Global Health in Otolaryngology

Editors

JAMES E. SAUNDERS
SUSAN R. CORDES
MARK E. ZAFEREO

OTOLARYNGOLOGIC CLINICS OF NORTH AMERICA

www.oto.theclinics.com

Consulting Editor
SUJANA S. CHANDRASEKHAR

June 2018 • Volume 51 • Number 3

ELSEVIER

1600 John F. Kennedy Boulevard • Suite 1800 • Philadelphia, Pennsylvania, 19103-2899

http://www.oto.theclinics.com

OTOLARYNGOLOGIC CLINICS OF NORTH AMERICA Volume 51, Number 3
June 2018 ISSN 0030-6665, ISBN-13: 978-0-323-58409-8

Editor: Jessica McCool
Developmental Editor: Sara Watkins

Otolaryngologic Clinics of North America (ISSN 0030-6665) is published bimonthly by Elsevier, Inc., 360 Park Avenue South, New York, NY 10010-1710. Months of issue are February, April, June, August, October, and December. Business and Editorial Offices: 1600 John F. Kennedy Blvd., Suite 1800, Philadelphia, PA 19103-2899. Customer Service Office: 6277 Sea Harbor Drive, Orlando, FL 32887-4800. Periodicals postage paid at New York, NY and additional mailing offices. Subscription prices are $396.00 per year (US individuals), $835.00 per year (US institutions), $100.00 per year (US student/resident), $519.00 per year (Canadian individuals), $1058.00 per year (Canadian institutions), $556.00 per year (international individuals), $1058.00 per year (international institutions), $270.00 per year (international & Canadian student/resident). Foreign air speed delivery is included in all *Clinics*' subscription prices. All prices are subject to change without notice. **POSTMASTER:** Send address changes to *Otolaryngologic Clinics of North America*, Elsevier Health Sciences Division, Subscription Customer Service, 3251 Riverport Lane, Maryland Heights, MO 63043. **Telephone: 1-800-654-2452 (U.S. and Canada); 314-447-8871 (outside U.S. and Canada). Fax: 314-447-8029. E-mail: journalscustomerservice-usa@elsevier.com (for print support); journalsonlinesupport-usa@elsevier.com (for online support).**

Reprints. For copies of 100 or more of articles in this publication, please contact the Commercial Reprints Department, Elsevier Inc., 360 Park Avenue South, New York, NY 10010-1710. Tel.: 212-633-3874; Fax: 212-633-3820; E-mail: reprints@elsevier.com.

Otolaryngologic Clinics of North America is also published in Spanish by McGraw-Hill Interamericana Editores S.A., P.O. Box 5-237, 06500 Mexico D.F., Mexico.

Otolaryngologic Clinics of North America is covered in *MEDLINE/PubMed (Index Medicus), Current Contents/Clinical Medicine, Excerpta Medica, BIOSIS, Science Citation Index,* and *ISI/BIOMED.*

PROGRAM OBJECTIVE

The goal of the *Otolaryngologic Clinics of North America* is to provide information on the latest trends in patient management, the newest advances; and provide a sound basis for choosing treatment options in the field of otolaryngology.

LEARNING OBJECTIVES

Upon completion of this activity, participants will be able to:

1. Review evidence-based approaches to pediatric otolaryngology in the developing world.
2. Discuss educational resources for global health in otolaryngology.
3. Recognize treatment strategies for global hearing loss prevention.

ACCREDITATION

The Elsevier Office of Continuing Medical Education (EOCME) is accredited by the Accreditation Council for Continuing Medical Education (ACCME) to provide continuing medical education for physicians.

The EOCME designates this enduring material for a maximum of 15 *AMA PRA Category 1 Credit*(s)™. Physicians should claim only the credit commensurate with the extent of their participation in the activity.

All other health care professionals requesting continuing education credit for this enduring material will be issued a certificate of participation.

DISCLOSURE OF CONFLICTS OF INTEREST

The EOCME assesses conflict of interest with its instructors, faculty, planners, and other individuals who are in a position to control the content of CME activities. All relevant conflicts of interest that are identified are thoroughly vetted by EOCME for fair balance, scientific objectivity, and patient care recommendations. EOCME is committed to providing its learners with CME activities that promote improvements or quality in healthcare and not a specific proprietary business or a commercial interest.

The planning committee, staff, authors and editors listed below have identified no financial relationships or relationships to products or devices they or their spouse/life partner have with commercial interest related to the content of this CME activity:
Jacqueline Alvarado, MD; Ryan H. Belcher, MD; Clifford Scott Brown, MD; Shelly Chadha, MBBS, MSurgery (ENT), PhD (Public Health); Pankaj Chaturvedi, MS, FAIS, FICS, FACS, MNAMS; Alarcos Cieza, MSc (Psychology), PhD (Medical Psychology); Susan Cordes, MD; Louise Davies, MD, MS, FACS; Susan D. Emmett, MD, MPH; Johannes J. Fagan, MBChB, M.Med., FCS (ORL); Dana Goldenberg; David Goldenberg, MD; Steven L. Goudy, MD; Melyssa Hancock, MD; Kristen Helm; Michael Hoa, MD; George Richard Holt, MD, MSE, MPH, MABE, D Bioethics; Alison Kemp; Miriam N. Lango, MD, FACS; Sonya MalekzAdeh, MD; Akshat Malik, MS, DNB; Anastasios Maniakas, MD; Adam Master, MD; Jessica McCool; Kevin Christopher McMains, MD; David W. Molter, MD; Eugene N. Myers, MD, FACS, FRCS Edin (Hon); Deepa Nair, MS, DNB, DORL; Kathryn Y. Noonan, MD; Randal A. Otto, MD; Zane Rankin, MPH; Kevin Thomas Robbins, MD; Samantha Kleindienst Robler, AuD, PhD; Sebastian Roesch, MD; Robert Saadi, MD; James E. Saunders, MD; David A. Shaye, MD; Hitesh Singhavi, MDS; James D. Smith, MD; Jose Pablo Stolovitzky, MD; Keng Lu Tan, MD; Debara L. Tucci, MD, MS, MBA, FACS; Subhalakshmi Vaidyanathan; Richard Wagner, MD; Brian D. Westerberg, MD, MHSc, FRCSC; Eric Wilkinson, MD; Gayle Woodson, MD; Mark E. Zafereo, MD, FACS.

The planning committee, staff, authors and editors listed below have identified financial relationships or relationships to products or devices they or their spouse/life partner have with commercial interest related to the content of this CME activity:
Regan W. Bergmark, MD: has received research support from American Board of Medical Specialties and the Gliklich Healthcare Innovation Scholar Grant. Dr. Bergmark's spouse has been a consultant/advisor with Janssen Pharmaceuticals, Inc and Daiichi Sankyo.
Mark G. Shrime, MD, PhD, MPH: owns stock in the GE Foundation and the Damon Runyon Cancer Research Foundation.
Maria V. Suurna, MD, FACS: has conducted clinical research sponsored by Inspire Medical Systems, Inc.

UNAPPROVED/OFF-LABEL USE DISCLOSURE

The EOCME requires CME faculty to disclose to the participants:

1. When products or procedures being discussed are off-label, unlabelled, experimental, and/or investigational (not US Food and Drug Administration [FDA] approved); and
2. Any limitations on the information presented, such as data that are preliminary or that represent ongoing research, interim analyses, and/or unsupported opinions. Faculty may discuss information about

pharmaceutical agents that is outside of FDA-approved labelling. This information is intended solely for CME and is not intended to promote off-label use of these medications. If you have any questions, contact the medical affairs department of the manufacturer for the most recent prescribing information.

TO ENROLL
To enroll in the *Otolaryngologic Clinics of North America* Continuing Medical Education program, call customer service at 1-800-654-2452 or sign up online at http://www.theclinics.com/home/cme. The CME program is available to subscribers for an additional annual fee of USD 260.

METHOD OF PARTICIPATION
In order to claim credit, participants must complete the following:
1. Complete enrolment as indicated above.
2. Read the activity.
3. Complete the CME Test and Evaluation. Participants must achieve a score of 70% on the test. All CME Tests and Evaluations must be completed online.

CME INQUIRIES/SPECIAL NEEDS
For all CME inquiries or special needs, please contact elsevierCME@elsevier.com.

Contributors

CONSULTING EDITOR

SUJANA S. CHANDRASEKHAR, MD
Past President, American Academy of Otolaryngology–Head and Neck Surgery, Partner, ENT & Allergy Associates, LLP, Clinical Professor, Department of Otolaryngology–Head and Neck Surgery, Zucker School of Medicine at Hofstra-Northwell, Hempstead, New York, USA; Clinical Associate Professor, Department of Otolaryngology–Head and Neck Surgery, Icahn School of Medicine at Mount Sinai, New York, New York, USA

EDITORS

JAMES E. SAUNDERS, MD, FACS
Professor, Otology and Neurotology, Department of Surgery, Dartmouth-Hitchcock Medical Center, Co-Chair, Coalition for Global Hearing Health, Senior Medical Director, Mayflower Medical Outreach, Lebanon, New Hampshire, USA

SUSAN R. CORDES, MD, FACS
Professor (Volunteer), Department of Surgery, Indiana University School of Medicine, Indianapolis, Indiana, USA; Department of Otolaryngology–Head and Neck Surgery, Adventist Health Ukiah Valley, Ukiah, California, USA

MARK E. ZAFEREO, MD, FACS
Associate Professor, Department of Head and Neck Surgery, Division of Surgery, Section Chief, Head and Neck Endocrine Surgery, The University of Texas MD Anderson Cancer Center, Houston, Texas, USA

AUTHORS

JACQUELINE ALVARADO, MD
Secretary, Pan-American Society of Otorhinolaryngology–Head and Neck Surgery, Atlanta, Georgia, USA; Past President, Venezuelan Society of Otolaryngology, Caracas, Venezuela

RYAN H. BELCHER, MD
Resident Physician, Department of Otolaryngology–Head and Neck Surgery, Emory University, Atlanta, Georgia, USA

REGAN W. BERGMARK, MD
Gliklich Healthcare Innovation Scholar, Department of Otolaryngology, Massachusetts Eye and Ear Infirmary, Harvard Medical School, Boston, Massachusetts, USA

CLIFFORD SCOTT BROWN, MD
Resident Physician, Department of Surgery, Division of Head and Neck Surgery & Communication Sciences, Duke University Medical Center, Durham, North Carolina, USA

SHELLY CHADHA, MBBS, MSurgery (ENT), PhD (Public Health)
WHO Department for Management of NCDs, Disability, Violence and Injury Prevention, World Health Organization, Geneva, Switzerland

PANKAJ CHATURVEDI, MS, FAIS, FICS, FACS, MNAMS
Professor, Head and Neck Surgical Oncology, Tata Memorial Centre, Mumbai, India

ALARCOS CIEZA, MSc (Psychology), PhD (Medical Psychology)
WHO Department for Management of NCDs, Disability, Violence and Injury Prevention, World Health Organization, Geneva, Switzerland

SUSAN R. CORDES, MD, FACS
Professor (Volunteer), Department of Surgery, Indiana University School of Medicine, Indianapolis, Indiana, USA; Department of Otolaryngology–Head and Neck Surgery, Adventist Health Ukiah Valley, Ukiah, California, USA

LOUISE DAVIES, MD, MS, FACS
Associate Professor of Surgery-Otolaryngology, Dartmouth Geisel School of Medicine, Hanover, New Hampshire, USA

SUSAN D. EMMETT, MD, MPH
Assistant Professor of Surgery and Global Health, Department of Surgery, Division of Head and Neck Surgery & Communication Sciences, Duke University Medical Center, Duke Global Health Institute, Durham, North Carolina, USA

JOHANNES J. FAGAN, MBChB, M.Med., FCS (ORL)
Professor and Chairman, Division of Otorhinolaryngology, Faculty of Health Sciences, University of Cape Town, Cape Town, South Africa

DANA GOLDENBERG
Tulane University, New Orleans, Louisiana, USA

DAVID GOLDENBERG, MD, FACS
Department of Surgery, Division of Otolaryngology–Head and Neck Surgery, Pennsylvania State University College of Medicine, Hershey, Pennsylvania, USA

STEVEN L. GOUDY, MD
Associate Professor of Pediatric Otolaryngology–Head and Neck Surgery, Emory University, Atlanta, Georgia, USA

MELYSSA HANCOCK, MD
Resident, Department of Otolaryngology–Head and Neck Surgery, Georgetown MedStar Hospital, Washington, DC, USA

MICHAEL HOA, MD
Assistant Professor, Department of Otolaryngology–Head and Neck Surgery, MedStar Georgetown University Hospital, Washington, DC, USA

GEORGE RICHARD HOLT, MD, MSE, MPH, MABE, D Bioethics
Professor, Department of Otolaryngology–Head and Neck Surgery, The University of Texas Health Science Center, San Antonio, Texas, USA

MIRIAM N. LANGO, MD, FACS
Associate Professor, Department of Surgical Oncology, Head and Neck Surgery Section, Fox Chase Cancer Center, Department of Otolaryngology, Temple University School of Medicine, Temple University Health System, Philadelphia, Pennsylvania, USA

SONYA MALEKZADEH, MD
Professor, Department of Otolaryngology–Head and Neck Surgery, MedStar Georgetown University Hospital, Washington, DC, USA

AKSHAT MALIK, MS, DNB
MCh Student, Head and Neck Surgical Oncology, Tata Memorial Centre, Mumbai, India

ANASTASIOS MANIAKAS, MD
Resident, Department of Surgery, Division of Otolaryngology–Head and Neck Surgery, Université de Montréal, Montreal, Québec, Canada

ADAM MASTER, MD
Fellow, Department of Otolaryngology–Head and Neck Surgery, House Ear Clinic, Divisions of Otology, Neurotology and Skull Base Surgery, University of California, Los Angeles, Los Angeles, California, USA

KEVIN CHRISTOPHER McMAINS, MD
Chief, Division of Otolaryngology–Head and Neck Surgery, Audie L. Murphy VA Medical Center, San Antonio, Texas, USA

DAVID W. MOLTER, MD
Professor of Pediatric Otolaryngology–Head and Neck Surgery, Washington University School of Medicine in St. Louis, St Louis, Missouri, USA

EUGENE N. MYERS, MD, FACS, FRCS Edin (Hon)
Distinguished Professor and Emeritus Chair, Department of Otolaryngology, University of Pittsburgh School of Medicine, Pittsburgh, Pennsylvania, USA

DEEPA NAIR, MS, DNB, DORL
Associate Professor, Head and Neck Surgical Oncology, Tata Memorial Centre, Mumbai, India

KATHRYN Y. NOONAN, MD
Fellow, House Ear Clinic, Los Angeles, California, USA

RANDAL A. OTTO, MD
Professor, Department of Otolaryngology–Head and Neck Surgery, The University of Texas Health Science Center, San Antonio, Texas, USA

ZANE RANKIN, MPH
Researcher, Institute for Health Metrics and Evaluation, Seattle, Washington, USA

KEVIN THOMAS ROBBINS, MD
Professor Emeritus, Southern Illinois University, Merritt Island, Florida, USA

SAMANTHA KLEINDIENST ROBLER, AuD, PhD
Director of Audiology, Norton Sound Health Corporation, Norton Sound Health, Nome, Alaska, USA

SEBASTIAN ROESCH, MD
Department of Otorhinolaryngology, Head and Neck Surgery, Paracelsus Medical University, Salzburg, Austria

ROBERT SAADI, MD
Department of Surgery, Division of Otolaryngology–Head and Neck Surgery, Pennsylvania State University College of Medicine, Hershey, Pennsylvania, USA

JAMES E. SAUNDERS, MD, FACS
Professor, Otology and Neurotology, Department of Surgery, Dartmouth-Hitchcock Medical Center, Co-Chair, Coalition for Global Hearing Health, Senior Medical Director, Mayflower Medical Outreach, Lebanon, New Hampshire, USA

DAVID A. SHAYE, MD
Instructor, Department of Otolaryngology, Massachusetts Eye and Ear Infirmary, Department of Global Health and Social Medicine, Program in Global Surgery and Social Change, Harvard Medical School, Boston, Massachusetts, USA; Associate Head, Department of Otolaryngology, University Teaching Hospital of Kigali, Rwanda

MARK G. SHRIME, MD, PhD, MPH
Assistant Professor, Department of Otolaryngology, Massachusetts Eye and Ear Infirmary, Director of Research, Program in Global Surgery and Social Change, Department of Global Health and Social Medicine, Harvard Medical School, Boston, Massachusetts, USA

HITESH SINGHAVI, MDS
Research Fellow, Head and Neck Surgical Oncology, Tata Memorial Centre, Mumbai, India

JAMES D. SMITH, MD
Professor Emeritus, Department of Otolaryngology, Oregon Health & Science University, Portland, Oregon, USA; Visiting Professor, Department of Otolaryngology, National University of Singapore, Singapore, Singapore

JOSE PABLO STOLOVITZKY, MD
Adjunct Assistant Professor, Department of Otolaryngology, Emory University School of Medicine, CEO, ENT of Georgia North, Atlanta, Georgia, USA

MARIA V. SUURNA, MD, FACS
Assistant Professor, Department of Otolaryngology–Head and Neck Surgery, Weill Cornell Medicine, New York, New York, USA

KENG LU TAN, MD
Consultant Ear, Nose and Throat, Head and Neck Surgeon, Department of Otolaryngology, Ipoh Specialist Hospital, Ipoh, Perak, Malaysia

DEBARA L. TUCCI, MD, MS, MBA, FACS
Professor, Department of Surgery, Division of Head and Neck Surgery & Communication Sciences, Duke University Medical Center, Durham, North Carolina, USA

RICHARD WAGNER, MD
Director, Global ENT Outreach, Coupeville, Washington, USA

BRIAN D. WESTERBERG, MD, MHSc, FRCSC
Clinical Professor, Department of Surgery, Division of Otolaryngology–Head and Neck Surgery, B.C. Rotary Hearing and Balance Centre, Director, Branch for International Surgical Care, University of British Columbia, Vancouver, British Columbia, Canada

ERIC WILKINSON, MD
Partner, House Ear Clinic, Los Angeles, California, USA

GAYLE WOODSON, MD
Professor, University of Central Florida, Merritt Island, Florida, USA

MARK E. ZAFEREO, MD, FACS
Associate Professor, Department of Head and Neck Surgery, Division of Surgery, Section Chief, Head and Neck Endocrine Surgery, The University of Texas MD Anderson Cancer Center, Houston, Texas, USA

Contents

Surgeons in sub-Saharan Africa face challenges different from those in developed countries: extreme shortages of otolaryngologists, speech pathologists, and audiologists; lack of training opportunities; and a paucity of otolaryngology services aggravated by population growth and aging. In addition to common Western diseases, patients have otolaryngology complications related to the human immunodeficiency virus, tuberculosis, malaria, and trauma. Less than 5% of the population has access to timely, safe, affordable surgery; 29 of 52 African countries have no radiotherapy services. Discussion focuses on education and training, which can be achieved in several ways, some complimentary.

Latin America has significant disparities that make the region vulnerable in the delivery of health care. There is a need to plan comprehensive health care strategies that result in a more robust trained health care workforce, while improving the quality and efficiencies of tertiary public hospitals. This article introduces a survey conducted among otorhinolaryngology leaders in the region that identified the need to strengthen postgraduate programs. Although all countries in Latin America have at least one residency program, more otorhinolaryngology-trained specialists are necessary to address the workforce shortages that are present in about 50% of Latin American countries.

The Asia-Pacific region has 60% of the world's population. There is a huge variability in ethnic groups, geography, diseases, and income. The otolaryngology workforce depends on the number of medical graduates, training programs, scope of practice, and available employment. Training has been influenced by the British, Russian, and US training systems and by local influences and experience. Otolaryngologic diseases are similar to those seen in the United States but with ethnic and regional differences. There are opportunities for humanitarian service, but the most sustainable projects will include repetitive visits with transfer of knowledge.

Evaluating and providing global health assistance, humanitarian aid, and medical missions to Middle Eastern countries can be rewarding and challenging. A broad spectrum of financial capabilities supports effective health care delivery and infrastructure. Middle East tension can make obtaining a visa difficult. Personal safety considerations may hinder efforts to develop and carry out clinical and educational programs. Several Middle East countries have sophisticated and modern health care systems.

Medical education and specialty training compare with those of Western medicine. The Middle East has a proud heritage as the foundation of many fundamental and modern medical and surgical principles.

Following recent geopolitical events and unification of Europe, the European Union (EU) is currently confronted with health care workforce shortage and insufficient uniform access to quality care. Aging population, difficulties with physician retention, and mobility of health care professionals are thought to contribute to this problem. Because of the differences in medical education and residency curriculum across the European countries, there is a need for a standardized training and certification. Current government initiatives are geared toward developing common policies and programs across the EU countries to address health care access.

In North America, underserved and vulnerable populations experience poorer health outcomes despite greater per capita health care expenditures. Biological, behavioral, and socioeconomic factors lead to more advanced disease presentation that may necessitate disparate treatment. In addition, vulnerable populations are more likely to obtain care from low-volume providers and are more likely to receive inappropriate care. Disparities in care are exacerbated by the distribution of the physician workforce and limited participation by physicians in the care of vulnerable populations. Multipronged strategies are needed to ameliorate observed disparities in care.

OTOLARYNGOLOGIC CLINICS
OF NORTH AMERICA

ISSUE OF RELATED INTEREST

Pediatric Clinics of North America, August 2017 (Vol. 64, No. 4)
Global Infections and Child Health
James P. Nataro, *Editor*
Available at: http://www.pediatric.theclinics.com/

Foreword

Otolaryngology Around the World

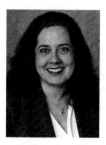

Sujana S. Chandrasekhar, MD
Consulting Editor

Humankind initially believed that the Earth was flat, and then, several centuries ago, mathematicians and astronomers proved that the Earth was round. As we complete the second decade of this century, we realize that, although the planet is spherical, the changing attitudes, free movement of people across borders, and access to ideas in all areas from cosmopolitan to rural sites, mean that the world is actually "flat." In his book, *The World Is Flat: A Brief History of the 21st Century,* Thomas Friedman alludes to the perceptual shift required for countries, companies, and individuals to remain competitive in a global market in which historical and geographic divisions have become increasingly irrelevant. How does this apply to Otolaryngology? Drs Saunders, Cordes, and Zafareo have compiled an extraordinarily thorough issue of *Otolaryngologic Clinics of North America* to show us just this.

In this issue of *Otolaryngologic Clinics of North America,* the reader is taken on a journey through the medical/surgical, economic, and cultural particulars of Otolaryngologic care around the world. As we know, quality of life is greatly enhanced by various otolaryngologic interventions. This is particularly important as the global burden of diseases of the ear, nose, and throat is high. Even in low-resource settings, technology can be utilized to bring the highest level of assessment and treatment to the patients, while staying practical regarding ongoing care and follow-up. Recognition by the World Health Organization of hearing loss as a major global health issue enables prevention, early identification, and treatment to curtail this problem. Diseases themselves manifest differently around the world, and it is necessary to be prepared for a different "normal" in different parts of the world; for example, in terms of goiter size, degree of involvement in suppurative otitis media, and extent of squamous cell carcinomas of the head and neck in various geographic settings. Two billion children live in the developing world, out of 2.2 billion children in total. Speech, language, and hearing disorders in these children, without proper recognition or treatment, can result in

Otolaryngol Clin N Am 51 (2018) xvii–xviii
https://doi.org/10.1016/j.otc.2018.02.003
0030-6665/18/© 2018 Published by Elsevier Inc.

oto.theclinics.com

life-long compromise. Applying evidence-based Otolaryngology care to these children will help to level that playing field as well.

Workforce needs must also be tailored to the local circumstances. I commend the Guest Editors of this compilation on providing in-depth analyses of workforce, training, and disease burdens in each of the following world areas: Africa, Latin America, Asia/Pacific, Middle East, Europe, and North America.

The smaller our world gets, and the easier communication becomes, the more it behooves health care professionals to understand the patterns of disease, of care, and of otolaryngology education in all areas. The Guest Editors of this issue of *Otolaryngology Clinics of North America*, Drs James Saunders, Susan Cordes, and Mark Zafareo, have brought their knowledge and experience in global ENT and have engaged likewise highly qualified authors to produce what is the authoritative reference on Global Health in Otolaryngology. I hope you enjoy exploring ENT around the world from the comfort of your armchair. I wouldn't be surprised if you are inspired to go abroad yourself!

Sujana S. Chandrasekhar, MD
ENT & Allergy Associates, LLP
18 East 48th Street, 2nd Floor
New York, NY 10017, USA

E-mail address:
ssc@nyotology.com

Preface

The Small World of Global Otolaryngology

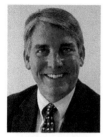   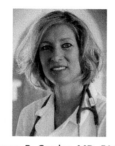   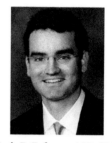

James E. Saunders, MD, FACS   Susan R. Cordes, MD, FACS   Mark E. Zafereo, MD, FACS
Editors

The world is indeed becoming smaller, and the medical field has been transformed by this rapid globalization. As global communication and travel have increased, the Otolaryngology-Head and Neck Surgery community has also become increasingly connected and interwoven across the world, from highly sophisticated tertiary care centers to rural communities in developing countries. As medical professionals, it has always been a part of our fiber to impart information and skills that improve the lives of patients; now, more than ever, it is incumbent upon physicians to share expertise on a global scale. The diseases treated by Otolaryngologists-Head and Neck Surgeons can differ widely in varying regions, but all can collaborate to learn from each other in order to advance the field and the care of patients around the world. To paraphrase the Global Health leaders Paul Farmer and Jim Kim, it is also incumbent upon Otolaryngologists to take a "view beyond the OR." In addition to providing care, we must consider the infrastructure that helps to support our patients and address the public health issues of disease screening and prevention.

We are proud to present this issue of *Otolaryngologic Clinics of North America* devoted to global Otolaryngology. We owe our deepest gratitude to the highly esteemed and experienced authors who have contributed their knowledge and expertise. This issue comprehensively addresses the global burden of Otolaryngology-Head and Neck Surgery Disease, evidence-based surgical and medical disease management, technology, and educational resources. A large emphasis is placed on Otolaryngology in low-resource settings, as this is clearly the area of greatest disparity and likewise greatest opportunity to improve patient care on a global scale. Additional articles delve more deeply into subspecialty care, including otology, head and neck surgery, and thyroid surgery. And finally, focused articles are dedicated to specific regions of the world, from Africa to Asia, from the Middle East to Europe, and from Latin America to North America. It is our hope and aspiration that the medical literature, readers,

Otolaryngol Clin N Am 51 (2018) xix–xx
https://doi.org/10.1016/j.otc.2018.02.002
0030-6665/18/© 2018 Published by Elsevier Inc.

and ultimately, and most importantly, patients, will benefit from continued mutual learning and collaborative global efforts in the field of Otolaryngology-Head and Neck Surgery.

James E. Saunders, MD, FACS
Otology & Neurotology
Department of Surgery
Dartmouth-Hitchcock Medical Center
Coalition for Global Hearing Health
Mayflower Medical Outreach
One Medical Center Drive
Lebanon, NH 03756, USA

Susan R. Cordes, MD, FACS
Department of Surgery
Indiana University
Indianapolis, IN, USA

Otolaryngology-Head and Neck Surgery
1165 South Dora Street, Suite C2
Adventist Health–Ukiah Valley
Ukiah, CA 95482, USA

Mark E. Zafereo, MD, FACS
Department of Head & Neck Surgery
Head & Neck Endocrine Surgery
MD Anderson Cancer Center
1515 Holcombe Boulevard, Unit 1445
Houston, TX 77030, USA

E-mail addresses:
james.saunders@hitchcock.org (J.E. Saunders)
susancordes@att.net (S.R. Cordes)
mzafereo@mdanderson.org (M.E. Zafereo)

Surgical Care and Otolaryngology in Global Health

Regan W. Bergmark, MD[a,b], David A. Shaye, MD[a,b,c,d],
Mark G. Shrime, MD, PhD, MPH[a,b,c,d],*

KEYWORDS

- Global health • Otolaryngology • Global surgery • Delivery of health care

KEY POINTS

- Surgical access is inadequate for most people; however, data on global surgery in general–global otolaryngology in particular–is limited because of a lack of studies with strong methodology.
- The Lancet Commission on Global Surgery established 6 indicators to measure surgical access: geographic accessibility, density of surgical providers, number of procedures performed, perioperative mortality, impoverishing expenditure, and catastrophic expenditure. Otolaryngology surgical, training, and research efforts use these 6 indicators to maximize impact and coordination of worldwide efforts in surgery.
- Research must be rigorous and consider the counterfactual: what would have happened had the intervention not taken place, confounders, and what else is happening at the time of the intervention.
- For otolaryngologists who want to contribute, focusing on 1 of the 6 indicators may be most impactful.

Disclosure Statement: The authors did not receive financial support specifically for this project, but all authors have academic research grant funding for their other work. R.W. Bergmark receives grant funding from the American Board of Medical Specialties Visiting Scholars Program and the Gliklich Healthcare Innovation Scholars Program. D. Shaye receives funding from Human Resources for Health - Rwandan Ministry of Health, a Foundation Grant from the AO Alliance, a Clinical Research Scholarship Grant from the American Academy of Facial Plastic and Reconstructive Surgery, and the Dubai Cooperative Research Grant from Harvard Medical School. M. Shrime receives funding from the Damon Runyon Cancer Research Foundation and the GE Foundation Safe Surgery 2020 Project.

[a] Department of Otolaryngology, Massachusetts Eye and Ear Infirmary, 243 Charles Street, Boston, MA 02114, USA; [b] Department of Otolaryngology, Harvard Medical School, 243 Charles Street, Boston, MA 02114, USA; [c] Department of Global Health and Social Medicine, Harvard Medical School, 641 Huntington Avenue, Boston, MA 02115, USA; [d] Program in Global Surgery and Social Change, Harvard Medical School, 641 Huntington Avenue, Boston, MA 02115, USA
* Corresponding author. Department of Otolaryngology, 243 Charles Street, Boston, MA 02114.
E-mail address: Shrime@mail.Harvard.edu

Otolaryngol Clin N Am 51 (2018) 501–513
https://doi.org/10.1016/j.otc.2018.01.001
0030-6665/18/

OPENING VIGNETTE

Sambany is a man in his 60s who worked as a rice farmer in Madagascar. He developed an enlarging neck mass over 30 years, which grew to twice the size of his head. He had sought medical attention at 10 different medical facilities, most of which lacked surgeons. The tumor, which had grown to 16 pounds, was eventually removed by surgeons on Mercy Ships, a case that received significant publicity.[1–3] Although the surgical care and postoperative care were free, the cost of the 2-day trip to get to receive care was so high that he had to sell his rice paddy to afford the transportation. Five people carried him on their backs for 2 days to get him to a road with a taxi, and then he endured a several-hour, expensive drive to get to the location of Mercy Ships. His surgery was successful, and he was eventually discharged home but had suffered catastrophic economic losses to arrive at treatment.

INTRODUCTION TO SURGICAL CARE IN GLOBAL HEALTH

At least 4.8 billion people do not have access to surgery worldwide.[4] Approximately 30% of the world's disease burden requires surgical decision-making,[5] and 81 million people are impoverished annually by the costs of surgery.[6] Nearly 17 million deaths are caused by surgical disease every year.[7] Meanwhile, only 6% of surgeries are performed in the poorest countries, accounting for a third of the world's population.[7] Global surgery, which is defined here as surgical care in low- and middle-income countries (LMICs), is a startlingly large field, covering most of the global population, most of the earth's land mass, and which cuts across all disease categories.[8] In spite of its magnitude, global surgery has often been referred to as the neglected stepchild of global health, due to a lack of attention to the problem.[9] Although charity efforts such as surgical mission trips in otolaryngology and surgery have taken place for decades in LMICs,[10] global surgery as a cohesive academic field is new. Attention was first given to surgical access in earnest in the 1990s, and rigorous research has only started as a substantial and coordinated effort in the last several years.[11] Several objectives have been prioritized:

1. Assessing needs on a global scale for surgical services to better define the problem and priorities
2. Standardizing benchmarks and outcome measures by which to measure surgical access
3. Finding and testing solutions to address the lack of surgical access, quality, affordability, and equity in LMICs

Lack of surgical care has actually grown in absolute numbers in LMICs, with any improvements unable to keep pace with improvements in other areas of health.[7] Barriers to surgical care include a scarcity of surgeons, anesthesiologists, and other staff; limited and poorly equipped facilities; limitations in ancillary services such as pathology and radiology; medication shortages and a dearth of operative equipment; and the high out-of-pocket cost of surgery. In one of the first large efforts to define the scope of surgical access problems globally in 2008, it was found that in sub-Saharan Africa, the density of operating rooms was just 1 per 100,000 people, compared with more than 14 per 100,000 in the United States.[12] Beneath this figure lie stark differences in quality and safety; up to 70% of operating rooms in sub-Saharan Africa are not even equipped with pulse oximetry.[12] It is estimated that from 2015 to 2030, the lack of access to effective, affordable, and safe surgery will result in $20.7 trillion in economic losses worldwide, with the economic losses disproportionately burdening poor countries.[13] Worldwide, 3.7 billion people are at risk catastrophic expenditure should they require surgery.[6] Surgical intervention has been shown to be cost-effective, saving major losses in productivity for patients.[13–17]

There are new global efforts to improve access to surgery worldwide. The World Health Organization's (WHO's) Safe Surgery Saves Lives initiative issued guidelines for surgical safety in 2009 as part of the WHO World Alliance for Patient Safety.[18] Further focus on the lack of access to surgical care worldwide prompted the Lancet Commission on Global Surgery (LCGS), launched in October 2013 and published in 2015. There is a new focus on the types of surgical platforms by which to improve access to surgical care, and in evaluating the efficacy of those interventions, as opposed to examining only the diseases treated.

Methodical and intensive efforts to address global surgery within the domain of otolaryngology are nascent. Only a few studies have systematically examined burden of otolaryngologic disease. For example, Van Buren and colleagues[19] completed a country-wide, cluster-randomized trial interviewing household members in Sierra Leone on the burden of head and neck disease. They found that 11.8% of patients suffered from a head and neck condition requiring evaluation for which they had not received medical care; 60.1% of patients cited cost as the reason why they had not sought care. Westerberg and colleagues[20] completed a cross-sectional study to evaluate the burden of otologic disease and hearing loss in Uganda, testing more than 6000 people with audiometric evaluation and otologic examination. They found that the prevalence of disabling hearing loss was 11.7% in adults and at least 10.3% of children.[20] More than 40% of children had obvious correctable causes of hearing loss with medical and surgical care.[20] These studies stand out as rarities for their rigor and size in determining the otolaryngology disease prevalence and surgical needs in low-income settings. Other studies have examined estimates of head and neck cancer prevalence by region,[21] or have built registries for specific conditions, such as with the Global Tracheostomy Collaborative.[22] Some people have studied case logs in LMIC as a way of looking at otolaryngology; while these data may illustrate presenting problems and the otolaryngology surgeries being performed, it may bear no resemblance to actual disease prevalence.[23] Data are limited within otolaryngology, and therefore much of the discussion here pertains to surgery at large in LMICs.

WHAT HAS MADE ACCESS TO SURGERY, INCLUDING OTOLARYNGOLOGY, SO CHALLENGING TO ADDRESS?

Global public health first developed in the fields of sanitation, nutrition, infectious disease, and communicable disease control. With the human immunodeficiency virus (HIV) epidemic for example, there was concerted worldwide effort to obtain reliable data on disease incidence and prevalence, find and treat at risk or infected patients, and objectively evaluate interventions using reproducible and rigorous methodology. The treatment of HIV, however, is different from the treatment of surgical disease. In HIV, a medication can be developed in a high-income country and brought, ready-made, to the country or region of need. In surgery, the corollary would be bringing the entire production line to the country in need.

The benefit of addressing surgical access–with its need to address factors from cost and equity to transportation systems, access to diagnostic testing, safe surgical theaters, blood banks, anesthesia care, sterilization, and training of surgeons and staff–is that the entire health care system must be improved to fix the surgical access problem. Potential exists for the development of significant positive externalities to the health system as a whole when focus is placed on surgery.

SUPPLY-SIDE BARRIERS TO SURGICAL CARE

Supply side barriers are defined by the inability of a health care system to offer safe, timely, accessible surgical care to its population. Many different resources are needed to provide surgical care: human resources including ancillary services, as well as equipment and medications.

Surgical Workforce

A lack of surgeons, anesthesiologists, obstetricians, nurses, radiologists, and pathologists or technicians in these fields has been a challenging barrier to improving access to surgical care. These problems are compounded by a lack of biomedical technicians and support and sterilization staff. The 80,000 otolaryngologists in the world are primarily in wealthy countries, with 2 orders of magnitude between the areas with the most and fewest otolaryngologists.[24] Addressing the surgical workforce crisis requires development and improvement of surgical training programs. Task shifting, such as providing surgical care by trained nonphysicians, is controversial but has been done successfully in some settings.[25]

Infrastructure

Lack of adequate surgical facilities and lack of equipment–such as surgical instruments, disposables such as suture or needles, and sterilization equipment–are common problems in LMICs. Medications may be unavailable in addition to monitoring equipment such as pulse oximetry in the operating room, ventilator support for ill patients, safe blood products, and a cold chain (refrigeration) for mediations requiring it. Infrastructure for ancillary services, such as microscopes and slide preparation materials for pathology or imaging equipment for radiology, also are included in infrastructure needs.

Quality of Service Delivery

Even with adequate human resources and infrastructure, quality surgical care requires a cohesive health care system that offers safe and affordable surgery. Quality surgical care depends on research that continuously evaluates surgical care, promoting an iterative process of improvement on what is being delivered.

DEMAND-SIDE BARRIERS TO SURGICAL CARE

Demand-side barriers are barriers that prevent patients from seeking medical attention. Even if surgical and medical services are robust, if demand for them is hampered, the health care system will continue to be dysfunctional.

Medical Costs

Both user fees at the time of arrival (such as copayments), as well as costs of medical and surgical care during or after treatment, can cause patients to delay or abandon attempts to seek medical attention. User fees, even if low, may prohibit a patient who can get to a hospital from being able to obtain care.[26] However, the impact of user fees on health care utilization and impoverishing or catastrophic health care expenditure for the patient is complex. In Uganda for example, user fees were abolished at governmental health facilities in 2001.[26] Although the use of these health care centers by the poor increased substantially at these sites, risk of catastrophic expenditure did not decrease. The authors hypothesized that this was because medications were scarce at government health facilities after 2001 and therefore needed to be purchased at private pharmacies. Additionally, there may have been informal payments—bribes—to health care providers. They recommended determining what the user fees fund and to take steps to ensure sustainability if they are going to be reduced or eliminated (eg, increasing public funding of health centers that will no longer be collecting user fees).[26,27] In Ethiopia, it was found that removal of user fees could paradoxically increase catastrophic expenditures for the poor while reducing catastrophic expenditures for the wealthy, because of these other expenses.[28]

Nonmedical Costs

Inadequate or costly transportation, costs of food and lodging, and the cost for caregivers all contribute additional economic barriers to patients even if medical care is free. Many countries or regions do not have any type of emergency travel or ambulance system, and have poor roads and infrastructure. In LMICs, physicians stated that the top barrier for their patients to seek medical or surgical care for cleft lip and palate, for example, was the cost of transport to a facility.[29] For Sambany (the patient in the opening vignette), the cost of transportation was catastrophic, even though the surgical care was actually free after he arrived for care.

Opportunity Costs

Loss of wages and inability to leave home because of family or home obligations also reduce demand for services.

Lack of Knowledge

Patients may be unaware that surgery or medical care can actually treat their condition, or unaware that such care is available, and therefore do not seek care.

Cultural Considerations

In some areas, patients do not seek care, because a family member does not want him or her traveling away from home (eg, "My husband won't let me go to the hospital").

Distrust and Fear

Fear or distrust of the medical system lowers demand for services.

Shame

Shame plays a particularly important role in stigmatizing diseases such as obstetric fistula[30] or cleft lip and palate.[31] In the case of the patient in the opening vignette, shame had kept him inside his home for many years before ultimately seeking care.

WORLD EFFORTS TO IMPROVE ACCESS TO SAFE, TIMELY, AND AFFORDABLE SURGERY

Several recent efforts have been made to understand and address the surgical disease burden worldwide. The Disease Control Priorities (DCP) program, the World Health Organization Safe Surgery Saves Lives Initiative, and the Lancet Commission on Global Surgery will be discussed.

Disease Control Priorities

The DCP program is managed by the University of Washington's Department of Global Health and the Institute for Health Metrics and Evaluation, and received funding from the Bill and Melinda Gates Foundation in 2009.[32] The DCP has made 3 major reports analyzing the global burden of disease as well as effectiveness of interventions, starting with DCP1 in 1993, DCP2 in 2006 (both published by the World Bank), and now the DCP3 which started in 2013. DCP3 provides data on cost-effectiveness, prioritization, and policy recommendations to prevent and treat the most pressing medical conditions.

The World Health Organization: Safe Surgery Saves Lives

WHO championed efforts to improve access to emergency and essential surgical care in the early 2000s. The next surgical initiative, the Safe Surgery Safe Lives Initiative, created a report published in 2009[18] as part of WHO's World Alliance for Patient Safety, which started in 2004.[33] The goals of the Safe Surgery Saves Lives Initiative included measuring surgical volume and basic outcomes data, preventing surgical site infections, improving teamwork in surgical teams, and improving the safety of anesthesia. The efforts included attempts at global implementation of a surgical safety checklist.

The Lancet Commission on Global Surgery: Six Indicators

The Lancet Commission on Global Surgery was convened with the goals of creating foundational research on global surgical access and quality, and galvanizing attention for global surgery. The commission brought together experts from across the world to define best approaches to the problem, a global needs assessment, and priorities for research and intervention. The commission's major report was published in April 2015.[7] The Lancet Commission on Global Surgery had 2 basic recommendations: the development of surgical plans for scaling up surgery at the national level, and standardization in the measurement and reporting of surgical access and quality. To the latter end, the Commission proposed 6 main surgical indicators with associated targets for 2030, which are presented in **Table 1**.[34]

Table 1
The Lancet Commission on Global Surgery 6 indicators

Indicator Name	Indicator Definition	2030 Target
1. Geographic access	The proportion of the population that can access a hospital capable of performing a cesarean section, a laparotomy, and an open fracture fixation within 2 h	80% of the population in each country with geographic access
2. Surgical workforce density	The number of surgeons, anesthesiologists and obstetrician-gynecologists per 100,000 people	At least 20 surgeons, anesthesiologists and obstetrician-gynecologists per 100,000 people
3. Surgical volume	The number of procedures per 100,000 people	At least 5000 procedures per 100,000 people; 100% of countries tracking surgical volume
4. Perioperative mortality rate	The mortality before discharge from the hospital	Measure and report perioperative mortality rate
5. Risk of impoverishing expenditure	The probability of being driven into or further into poverty because of costs of surgery	0% of people at risk of impoverishing expenditure
6. Risk of catastrophic expenditure	The probability of facing an expenditure of >10% of household income spent for surgery	0% of people at risk of catastrophic expenditure

Data from Meara JG, Leather AJ, Hagander L, et al. Global Surgery 2030: evidence and solutions for achieving health, welfare, and economic development. Lancet 2015;386(9993):569–624.

Ideally all indicators should be used together to avoid the unintended consequences of optimizing 1 indicator without attention to the others (eg, increasing surgical volume without attention to perioperative mortality). Given the scarcity of reliable data on surgical access in LMIC, evaluation by these 6 indicators provides a good estimate of surgical capacity and access in a given region, and should be responsive to change after an intervention is undertaken. The indicators have already been used in some countries such as Madagascar to identify areas of deficiency.[35] The data are also easily interpretable to governmental or nongovernmental agencies, and cover a wide array of surgical procedures and measures of capacity and staffing. Implementation tools, such as an in-depth description of the 6 indicators, a surgical assessment tool for a hospital walk-through evaluation (eg, to methodically determine and record the capacity of a hospital to provide critical services, anything from oxygen to blood draws), surveys to determine catastrophic and impoverishing expense, and examples of national surgical plans are publicly available.[34,36]

RESEARCH IN GLOBAL SURGERY: BEST APPROACHES

The World Health Organization has promoted a model for universal health coverage with financing decisions made along 3 axes: who in the population is covered, which services are covered, and the proportion of direct costs that are covered.[37] These 3 axes could be translated into the domains of (1) equity, (2) health, and (3) financial risk protection. Any evaluation of interventions in global surgery should take these 3 domains into account in measurement of outcomes and in prioritization of programs. For example, an intervention that improves health but with a high risk of catastrophic expenditure for patients, and which is only available to the nonpoor, would do poorly in 2 of the 3 domains. A ministry of health should be able to understand the implications of a specific intervention in terms of cost and equity as well as in terms of health.

Currently, research within global surgery in general and in global otolaryngology in particular is extremely limited, but increasing.[38] There are no randomized controlled trials in global otolaryngology to the authors' knowledge. Observational studies are generally small and plagued with selection bias. Preintervention and postintervention studies are most common, but that study design is flawed in that the counterfactual is ignored. Most otolaryngology research falls into this category, and relates to the number of procedures performed, manuscripts published, or otolaryngologists trained before and after an intervention is undertaken, without addressing the counterfactual including potential downsides of intervention.[23,39]

In the design of future research, general principles of ethics and research study design must be followed, regardless of whether the researcher is working in a high-income country or LMIC. Common errors such as the lack of a control group or ignoring confounders must be avoided. Without comparison to the counterfactual and without attention to confounders, it is not possible to know if the intervention caused improvement in a health care system (or harm), or if changes in the health care system would have occurred regardless of the intervention. Robust study designs such as cluster randomization, randomized trials, and modeling can all allow for methodologically sound data generation.

In addition to crafting a methodologically sound study, there are other aspects of international research that must be taken into account. As defined by the Lancet Commission, these include appropriateness of the study, local ownership and initiative for the project, authorship concerns (with the goal of projects being done by or including authors from the region in question), consent, and plans for the treatment of medically concerning conditions found during research.

MODELS FOR IMPACTING GLOBAL OTOLARYNGOLOGY AND SURGICAL CAPACITY

There are multiple platforms for improving surgical access and quality, which can be categorized based on the method they use to deliver care (rather than by specialty)[10] and include (1) governmental efforts; (2) nongovernmental efforts such as (2a) short term surgical trips, (2b) self-contained surgical platforms and (2c) surgical specialty hospitals; and (3) surgical training programs. Disaster relief, humanitarian emergency outreach programs, and research training programs are beyond the scope of this article.

This section will briefly describe each method of surgical care delivery as it pertains to global surgery at large in LMICs, with mention of otolaryngology where there is sufficient evidence base to do so.

Governmental Efforts

These efforts are generally led by the government and ministries of health and can include building, improving, or expanding existing hospitals and health care facilities, residency and staff training programs, public outreach and education, and infrastructure such as emergency response systems. Government efforts can also reduce costs to patients by reducing or eliminating user fees or providing vouchers for nonmedical costs.

Efforts by Nongovernmental Organizations

Nongovernmental organizations (NGOs) have helped to fill the gap in surgical services in LMICs. A study examining the role of NGOs in the provision of surgical care identified 403 NGOs through a Web search that provided surgical care, two-thirds of which provided surgical care using a mission model.[40] Most organizations provided surgical services in the context of other care, while 39% provided only surgical services; of these, most were specialty-specific.[40] Twenty-six of the 403 organizations were otolaryngology NGOs, and an additional 78 were organizations dedicated to cleft lip and palate surgery.[40] Approximately half of NGOs managed at least 1 hospital. General surgery, obstetrics and gynecology, and plastic surgery were the 3 most common categories of surgical care provided.[40] Nongovernmental efforts can be divided into three major categories (a) short term surgical trips, (b) self-contained surgical platforms and (c) surgical specialty hospitals.[10]

Temporary surgical platforms: short term surgical trips (mission trips)

The surgical mission model is the most common form of involvement of otolaryngologists in global surgery efforts in LMICs, with 67% of NGOs using this model,[40] although most partnerships or trips do not result in published or publically available data for evaluation of efficacy. Evidence of benefit in the literature predominantly shows benefit for surgical trainees from the sending institutions (for example, institutions in the United States, Europe, Canada, or Australia)[41,42] rather than for the patient population in question or surgical trainees within LMICs. Mission models sometimes have a component of training as a goal but generally focus more on surgical output.[43] Research on mission models is sparse but generally defines success as cases completed, possibly with follow up, without controlling for factors such as resource utilization, displacement of local surgeons, disruption of the local medical economy, and negative unintended consequences (eg, using 2 operating rooms and limiting the other types of surgeries a facility can perform while the intervention is taking place). Outcomes for surgeons on surgical missions can be much worse than in their home institution and in fact no better than those of local surgeons, often attributed to factors such as health care and referral systems, patient age, nutrition, and other factors that the mission model does not generally correct.[44]

Temporary surgical platforms: self-contained surgical platforms

Self-contained surgical platforms, such as the US Navy hospital ships, Mercy Ships, CinterAndes, or Orbis, tend to stay in a region for a longer period of time but bring all needed infrastructure with them. These platforms are much more rare than the standard mission model. They usually provide a larger array of surgical services with greater long-term follow-up, but when they leave, frequently depart without leaving any significant health care infrastructure behind. Self-contained platforms may be particularly useful in disaster scenarios.

Nongovernmental organization surgical specialty hospitals

Some NGOs have established stand-alone hospitals, or sections of hospitals. These specialty centers are generally dedicated to a single type of surgical intervention, such as eye surgery at the Aravind Eye Hospital, or the Guwahati Comprehensive Cleft Care Center.[45]

Surgical Training Programs

Surgical training programs, such as starting or supporting a residency training program or the training of surgeons or surgical practitioners, has been a focus of a scattering of otolaryngology and broader surgical efforts. For example, the University of Cape Town Karl Storz Head and Neck Surgery Fellowship in South Africa was the first head and neck cancer fellowship in sub-Saharan Africa, modeled on US fellowship programs, and has trained more than 10 surgeons who have all returned to their countries of origin within sub-Saharan Africa to lead and develop head and neck cancer services.[46] In addition, those surgeons have led 1- to 2-week training courses for other African otolaryngologists.[47,48] Isaacson has written about the challenges of developing a residency program in Ethiopia.[49] Ultimately, surgical training is based on an apprenticeship model that requires sustained and consistent effort and investment from experienced surgeons. Short-term models, in which residents in the host country witness complex surgeries without taking a leading role and without a long-term relationship with the teacher, are likely of little value.[49]

Other efforts are national and cross specialties. In Rwanda for example, the Human Resources for Health model was started in 2012 and brings seasoned surgeons and other physicians from the United States to Rwanda for several months to years.[50–53] These physicians then work with Rwandan surgeons to facilitate training. In a survey study of Rwandan and US physicians who participated in this program, 52% of Rwandan physicians but only 10% of US physicians felt that this twinning model had facilitated skill transfer effectively.[52] Only 38% of Rwandan physicians and 28% of US physicians said they were very satisfied with the model.[52]

Academic partnerships between sister institutions (eg, between an academic medical center in a high income country and one in an LMIC) have been popular within otolaryngology and across surgical fields, although there is limited research on efficacy.[54] More research is needed, as current research shows an increased number of trainees and publications,[55] but without an adequate control group. These partnerships may have multiple goals, including research, to offer trainees from high-income countries a more diverse operative experience in LMICs, and to train LMIC surgeons.[56]

The evidence base for teaching models and surgical workforce development is weak; further research is needed. Surgical training interventions rarely compare their results with a state of nonintervention, such that it is difficult to discern if any potential improvement would have naturally occurred without the intervention. Long-term follow-up to determine important outcomes such as staff retention, patient outcomes, and surgical volume is also needed.

NEXT STEPS FOR OTOLARYNGOLOGY

The framework created in the past several years for global surgery should be leveraged by otolaryngology. The authors propose several priorities.

Utilizing the Lancet Commission for Global Surgery six indicators should be utilized and built upon in efforts to define the otolaryngology disease burden and access to surgical care. Strong research done well is sorely lacking, making it difficult to measure the impact of interventions. Country-specific data in particular are greatly needed.[57]

Current work in otolaryngology, including partnerships, training models, and areas of greatest need should be catalogued. Some of these efforts are happening regionally, to create training program databases.[58]

Ethical guidelines for international involvement in otolaryngology surgical care, teaching, and research should be developed. For example, there have already been extensive discussions about resident involvement in overseas mission trips. As interest in global otolaryngology continues to grow, a framework for ethically and soundly approaching global otolaryngology would be helpful. Any ethical considerations must be made in conjunction with partners in LMICs.

Ongoing efforts to include global otolaryngology in policy and discussion within national otolaryngology societies should be nurtured.[59]

Best ways to offer cost-effective surgery and technologies for otolaryngologic conditions, based on disease burden and national priorities in LMICs should be determined.[60]

Otolaryngologists should shift their ongoing international involvement from short-term isolated volunteer trips, to research, training, and local partnerships that will impact the 6 Lancet Commission indicators. For example, an otolaryngologist working on surgical safety in the United States can apply his or her expertise in a resource-poor setting. If efforts are applied toward a common cause, the impact on patients in the poorest regions of the world will be magnified. With 70% of the world population unable to access timely, safe, and affordable surgery, there is moral imperative to embrace these concerted and cohesive efforts to impact surgical services at unprecedented scale.

REFERENCES

1. Shrime M, Meara J. How surgery can fight global poverty. The New York Times 2015.
2. Volunteer doctors remove facial tumour twice the size of Madagascan man's head. ABC News 2015.
3. Shrime MG. The right to look human-head and neck surgery in low- and middle-income countries: the Chris O'Brien Memorial Lecture. JAMA Otolaryngol Head Neck Surg 2016;142(12):1143–4.
4. Alkire BC, Raykar NP, Shrime MG, et al. Global access to surgical care: a modelling study. Lancet Glob Health 2015;3(6):e316–23.
5. Shrime MG, Bickler SW, Alkire BC, et al. Global burden of surgical disease: an estimation from the provider perspective. Lancet Glob Health 2015;3(Suppl 2):S8–9.
6. Shrime MG, Dare AJ, Alkire BC, et al. Catastrophic expenditure to pay for surgery worldwide: a modelling study. Lancet Glob Health 2015;3(Suppl 2):S38–44.

7. Meara JG, Leather AJ, Hagander L, et al. Global Surgery 2030: evidence and solutions for achieving health, welfare, and economic development. Lancet 2015; 386(9993):569–624.
8. Bickler SW, Spiegel D. Improving surgical care in low- and middle-income countries: a pivotal role for the World Health Organization. World J Surg 2010;34(3):386–90.
9. Farmer PE, Kim JY. Surgery and global health: a view from beyond the OR. World J Surg 2008;32(4):533–6.
10. Shrime MG, Sleemi A, Ravilla TD. Charitable platforms in global surgery: a systematic review of their effectiveness, cost-effectiveness, sustainability, and role training. World J Surg 2015;39(1):10–20.
11. Mock CN, Donkor P, Gawande A, et al. Essential surgery: key messages of this volume. In: Debas HT, Donkor P, Gawande A, et al, editors. Essential surgery: disease control priorities, third edition, vol. 1. Washington, DC: The International Bank for Reconstruction and Development/The World Bank (c) 2015 International Bank for Reconstruction and Development/The World Bank; 2015. p. 1–18.
12. Funk LM, Weiser TG, Berry WR, et al. Global operating theatre distribution and pulse oximetry supply: an estimation from reported data. Lancet 2010; 376(9746):1055–61.
13. Alkire BC, Shrime MG, Dare AJ, et al. Global economic consequences of selected surgical diseases: a modelling study. Lancet Glob Health 2015;3(Suppl 2):S21–7.
14. Alkire BC, Vincent JR, Meara JG. Benefit-cost analysis for selected surgical interventions in low- and middle-income countries. In: Debas HT, Donkor P, Gawande A, et al, editors. Essential surgery: disease control priorities, third edition, vol. 1. Washington, DC: The International Bank for Reconstruction and Development/The World Bank (c) 2015 International Bank for Reconstruction and Development/The World Bank; 2015. p. 361–80.
15. Chao TE, Sharma K, Mandigo M, et al. Cost-effectiveness of surgery and its policy implications for global health: a systematic review and analysis. Lancet Glob Health 2014;2(6):e334–45.
16. Corlew DS, Alkire BC, Poenaru D, et al. Economic valuation of the impact of a large surgical charity using the value of lost welfare approach. BMJ Glob Health 2016;1(4):e000059.
17. Grimes CE, Henry JA, Maraka J, et al. Cost-effectiveness of surgery in low- and middle-income countries: a systematic review. World J Surg 2014;38(1):252–63.
18. WHO Guidelines Approved by the Guidelines Review Committee. WHO guidelines for safe surgery 2009: safe surgery saves lives. Geneva (Switzerland): World Health Organization; 2009.
19. Van Buren NC, Groen RS, Kushner AL, et al. Untreated head and neck surgical disease in Sierra Leone: a cross-sectional, countrywide survey. Otolaryngol Head Neck Surg 2014;151(4):638–45.
20. Westerberg BD, Lee PK, Lukwago L, et al. Cross-sectional survey of hearing impairment and ear disease in Uganda. J Otolaryngol Head Neck Surg 2008;37(6):753–8.
21. Hussein AA, Helder MN, de Visscher JG, et al. Global incidence of oral and oropharynx cancer in patients younger than 45 years versus older patients: a systematic review. Eur J Cancer 2017;82:115–27.
22. Lavin J, Shah R, Greenlick H, et al. The Global Tracheostomy Collaborative: one institution's experience with a new quality improvement initiative. Int J Pediatr Otorhinolaryngol 2016;80:106–8.
23. Kligerman MP, Alexandre A, Jean-Gilles P, et al. Otorhinolaryngology/head and neck surgery in a low income country: the Haitian experience. Int J Pediatr Otorhinolaryngol 2017;93:128–32.

24. Alberti PW. Pediatric ear, nose and throat services' demands and resources: a global perspective. Int J Pediatr Otorhinolaryngol 1999;49(Suppl 1):S1–9.

25. Shrime MG, Sekidde S, Linden A, et al. Sustainable development in surgery: the health, poverty, and equity impacts of charitable surgery in Uganda. PLoS One 2016;11(12):e0168867.

26. Xu K, Evans DB, Kadama P, et al. Understanding the impact of eliminating user fees: utilization and catastrophic health expenditures in Uganda. Soc Sci Med 2006;62(4):866–76.

27. James CD, Hanson K, McPake B, et al. To retain or remove user fees?: reflections on the current debate in low- and middle-income countries. Appl Health Econ Health Policy 2006;5(3):137–53.

28. Shrime MG, Verguet S, Johansson KA, et al. Task-sharing or public finance for the expansion of surgical access in rural Ethiopia: an extended cost-effectiveness analysis. Health Policy Plan 2016;31(6):706–16.

29. Massenburg BB, Jenny HE, Saluja S, et al. Barriers to cleft lip and palate repair around the world. J Craniofac Surg 2016;27(7):1741–5.

30. Mwini-Nyaledzigbor PP, Agana AA, Pilkington FB. Lived experiences of Ghanaian women with obstetric fistula. Health Care Women Int 2013;34(6):440–60.

31. Mzezewa S, Muchemwa FC. Reaction to the birth of a child with cleft lip or cleft palate in Zimbabwe. Trop Doct 2010;40(3):138–40.

32. (DCP) -3 DCP. About the Project. 2017. Available at: http://dcp-3.org/about-project. Accessed July 21, 2017.

33. The World Alliance for Patient Safety at the World Health Organization. The second global patient safety challenge: safe surgery saves lives. Geneva (Switzerland): World Health Organization; 2008.

34. The Lancet Commission on Global Surgery. Implementation tools. Available at: http://www.lancetglobalsurgery.org/implementation-tools. Accessed July 30, 2017.

35. Bruno E, White MC, Baxter LS, et al. An evaluation of preparedness, delivery and impact of surgical and anesthesia care in Madagascar: a framework for a national surgical plan. World J Surg 2017;41(5):1218–24.

36. Change PiGSaS. National surgical, obstetric and anesthesia planning. 2017; Available at: www.pgssc.org/national-surgical-planning. Accessed July 21, 2017.

37. Organization WH. Universal coverage - three dimensions. Health financing for universal coverage 2017; Available at: www.who.int/health_financing/strategy/dimensions/en. Accessed July 21, 2017.

38. Chambers KJ, Creighton F, Abdul-Aziz D, et al. Global health-related publications in otolaryngology are increasing. Laryngoscope 2015;125(4):848–51.

39. Byaruhanga R, Rourke R, Awubwa M, et al. Increased frequency of visits improves the efficiency of surgical global health initiatives. J Otolaryngol Head Neck Surg 2013;42:41.

40. Ng-Kamstra JS, Riesel JN, Arya S, et al. Surgical non-governmental organizations: global surgery's unknown nonprofit sector. World J Surg 2016;40(8):1823–41.

41. Jafari A, Tringale KR, Campbell BH, et al. Impact of humanitarian experiences on otolaryngology trainees: a follow-up study of travel grant recipients. Otolaryngol Head Neck Surg 2017;156(6):1084–7.

42. Kelly K, McCarthy A, McLean L. Distributed learning or medical tourism? A Canadian residency program's experience in global health. J Surg Educ 2015;72(4):e33–45.

43. Boston M, Horlbeck D. Humanitarian surgical missions: planning for success. Otolaryngol Head Neck Surg 2015;153(3):320–5.

44. Maine RG, Hoffman WY, Palacios-Martinez JH, et al. Comparison of fistula rates after palatoplasty for international and local surgeons on surgical missions in Ecuador with rates at a craniofacial center in the United States. Plast Reconstr Surg 2012;129(2):319e–26e.

45. Campbell A, Restrepo C, Mackay D, et al. Scalable, sustainable cost-effective surgical care: a model for safety and quality in the developing world, part III: impact and sustainability. J Craniofac Surg 2014;25(5):1685–9.

46. Aswani J, Baidoo K, Otiti J. Establishing a head and neck unit in a developing country. J Laryngol Otol 2012;126(6):552–5.

47. Chambers KJ, Aswani J, Patel A, et al. The value of a collaborative course for advanced head and neck surgery in East Africa. Laryngoscope 2015;125(4): 883–7.

48. Fagan JJ, Aswani J, Otiti J, et al. Educational workshops with graduates of the University of Cape Town Karl Storz Head and Neck Surgery Fellowship Program: a model for collaboration in outreach to developing countries. Springerplus 2016; 5(1):1652.

49. Isaacson G. Framework for advancing otolaryngology: head and neck surgery in Ethiopia. Otolaryngol Head Neck Surg 2014;151(4):634–7.

50. Binagwaho A, Farmer PE. The human resources for health program in Rwanda. N Engl J Med 2014;370(10):981–2.

51. Shelton JD, Hodgins S. The human resources for health program in Rwanda. N Engl J Med 2014;370(10):981.

52. Ndenga E, Uwizeye G, Thomson DR, et al. Assessing the twinning model in the Rwandan Human Resources for Health Program: goal setting, satisfaction and perceived skill transfer. Glob Health 2016;12:4.

53. Cancedda C, Riviello R, Wilson K, et al. Building workforce capacity abroad while strengthening global health programs at home: participation of seven Harvard-affiliated institutions in a health professional training initiative in Rwanda. Acad Med 2017;92(5):649–58.

54. DeGennaro VA Jr, DeGennaro VA, Kochhar A, et al. Accelerating surgical training and reducing the burden of surgical disease in Haiti before and after the earthquake. J Craniofac Surg 2012;23(7 Suppl 1):2028–32.

55. Lipnick M, Mijumbi C, Dubowitz G, et al. Surgery and anesthesia capacity-building in resource-poor settings: description of an ongoing academic partnership in Uganda. World J Surg 2013;37(3):488–97.

56. Bergmark R, Williams W, Riesel JN, et al. Developing surgical capacity: models of implementation. In: Meara JG, McClain CD, Rogers SO, et al, editors. Global surgery and anesthesia manual, providing care in resource-limited settings. Boca Raton (FL): CRC Press; 2014.

57. Fuller JC, Shaye DA. Global surgery: current evidence for improving surgical care. Curr Opin Otolaryngol Head Neck Surg 2017;25(4):300–6.

58. Fagan JJ, Jacobs M. Survey of ENT services in Africa: need for a comprehensive intervention. Glob Health Action 2009. [Epub ahead of print].

59. Koch WM. 2009 American Head and Neck Society presidential address: going global, reaching out. Arch Otolaryngol Head Neck Surg 2009;135(11):1074–6.

60. Emmett SD, Tucci DL, Smith M, et al. GDP Matters: cost effectiveness of cochlear implantation and deaf education in Sub-Saharan Africa. Otol Neurotol 2015;36(8): 1357–65.

Otolaryngology and the Global Burden of Disease

James E. Saunders, MD[a],*, Zane Rankin, MPH[b], Kathryn Y. Noonan, MD[c]

KEYWORDS

- Global Burden of Disease • Disability-adjusted life years (DALY)
- Years lived with disease (LYD) • Hearing loss

KEY POINTS

- The Global Burden of Disease (GBD) project analyzes the comparative burden of all diseases to allow for appropriate allocation of health resources.
- GBD measures the all-cause mortality, years of life lost, the years of life lived with disability (YLD), and the combination of these in the disability-adjusted life years (DALYs) for multiple causes.
- The global burden of hearing loss is broken down into the sequelae of otitis media, meningitis, congenital causes, and to an age-related and other category.
- Hearing loss accounts for a significant disease burden globally with global YLDs comparable with diabetes and DALYs comparable with tuberculosis.
- Longitudinal data show a decrease in the incidence of head and neck cancers; however, thyroid cancer has become more prevalent without a corresponding increase in DALYs.

INTRODUCTION AND RELEVANCE TO OTOLARYNGOLOGY

The Global Burden of Disease (GBD) project provides a framework for analyzing the comparative burden of all diseases to allow for appropriate allocation of health resources. Measuring otolaryngologic contributions to the global burden of disease allows us to quantify the magnitude of health loss from these pathologies. Through the work of the GBD, there is a growing recognition that noncommunicable and surgical diseases, such as cancer and trauma, have a large impact on global health. This article introduces the basic methodology of the GBD and highlights the impact of this work on specific otolaryngologic conditions, such as hearing loss, otitis media, cleft lip and palate, head and neck cancer, oral disorders, and trauma.

Disclosure: The authors have nothing to disclose.
[a] Geisel Medical School at Dartmouth, Dartmouth Hitchcock Medical Center, One Medical Center Drive, Lebanon, NH 03756, USA; [b] Institute for Health Metrics and Evaluation, 2301 Fifth Avenue, Suite 600, Seattle, WA 98121, USA; [c] House Ear Clinic, 2100 West 3rd Street, Los Angeles, CA 90057-1999, USA
* Corresponding author.
E-mail address: James.E.Saunders@hitchcock.org

GLOBAL BURDEN OF DISEASE OVERVIEW

The GBD project is currently managed by the Institute for Health Metrics and Evaluation (IHME) at the University of Washington. The goal of GBD is to objectively and independently estimate the morbidity and mortality of all major causes of health loss. The GBD uses descriptive epidemiologic analyses to compare the effects of different diseases, injuries, and risk factors across a comprehensive set of age, sex, and locations. Such comparisons allow health policy decision-makers an opportunity to see the major contributors to health loss in a given sector. The GBD does this by estimating the all-cause mortality, deaths by cause, years of life lost (YLLs) due to premature mortality, years lived with disability (YLDs), and disability-adjusted life years (DALYs) for a specified list of disease causes (known as the *cause list*). These metrics are updated and recalculated annually as new information comes to light. Therefore, the most accurate estimates possible are available across a time span dating back to the original studies and publicized by the GBD (**Fig. 1**). The GBD has publicized these results through more than 270 scientific articles in the last 10 years as well as numerous policy reports, Web content, and open-access interactive visualizations (vizhub.healthdata.org/gbd-compare).[1]

The GBD estimates have an egalitarian ethos; the fundamental comparison used for mortality and morbidity, a healthy year of life, holds the same value in all countries. Mortality is measured in years lost from a global standard of highest observed life expectancy. The morbidity of conditions is quantified using disability weights shared by all countries. Using a life expectancy tied not to location but to the longest life span achieved by people acknowledges that, although geography holds an outsized influence on life expectancy and health outcomes, this should not be the case and we must work to eliminate health disparity. This goal sets a high bar for achievement in health improvement goals. The GBD estimation process is highly interconnected; each year new data and revised methods improve results in all sectors of burden estimation.

BACKGROUND AND GROWTH OF THE GLOBAL BURDEN OF DISEASE PROJECT

The GBD was originally founded by Drs Christopher Murray and Alan Lopez, who recognized in the early 1990s that the sum of deaths attributed to specific causes was greater than the total number of global deaths per year. In an effort to address this discrepancy, they began working on a more cohesive estimate of worldwide deaths as well as the impact of nonfatal health outcomes. Their initial study showed a substantial impact on health from such dissimilar problems as heart disease, road injuries, and depression.[2] They derived DALY to enable comparisons of the burden of disease, both in terms of life lost and disability of nonfatal outcomes. The first peer-reviewed GBD articles were published in 1997, and the World Health Organization established a Disease Burden Unit in 1998. The GBD 2010 study represented a landmark for 2 reasons: First, it was a truly collaborative effort engaging a worldwide network of 422 researchers. Second, GBD 2010 collaborators revised estimates for the 20-year interval from 1990 to 2010, replacing what had been a snapshot of global health with a quantitative narrative of health trends over time (see **Fig. 1**). Each rendition of the GBD includes new data sources, refined methodology, and a more comprehensive and detailed list of diseases and risk factors.[3] The methodology of the GBD has also been incorporated into numerous studies to compare the cost-effectiveness of different health strategies and treatments.

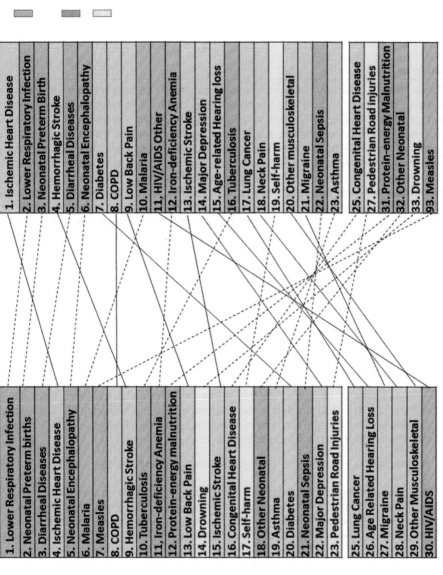

Fig. 1. Comparison of global GBD rank list based on DALYs for 1990 and 2015 (fourth hierarchy level causes for both sexes and all ages). COPD, chronic obstructive pulmonary disease; HIV, human immunodeficiency virus; inj, injury. (*Adapted from* Institute for Health Metrics and Evaluation (IHME). GBD compare. Seattle (WA): IHME, University of Washington; 2018. Available at: http://vizhub.healthdata.org/gbd-compare.)

BASIC GLOBAL BURDEN OF DISEASE METHODOLOGY AND TERMS

The 4 basic components of an estimate of the GBD are the all-cause mortality, causes of death, nonfatal outcomes, and risk factor analysis. These basic concepts are briefly discussed later. Cause of death estimates and nonfatal outcomes are combined into the signature measure of the GBD, the DALY.

All-Cause Mortality

All-cause mortality is defined as the mortality rate for a population across all causes. GBD all-cause mortality estimates are intended to be the most accurate estimates of death rates; therefore, it must equal the sum of cause-specific mortality. Unfortunately, many low- and middle-income countries lack robust vital registration systems, requiring sophisticated modeling to produce accurate mortality estimates.[1]

Causes of Death

Cause-specific mortality is fundamentally important knowledge; the rates and numbers of people who die of different diseases is critical to health policy planning and prioritizing research. Trends in causes of death also provide an important geographic summary of whether societies are making progress in reducing avoidable mortality.[4] For GBD, each death is attributed to a single underlying cause, the cause that initiated the series of events leading to death, in accordance with *International Classification of Diseases*. In estimating causes of death, the GBD study uses vital registration systems, mortality surveillance systems, censuses, surveys, police records, and verbal autopsies (surveys that collect information from individuals familiar with the deceased about the signs and symptoms the person had before death). After reconciling cause-specific death rates with the total all-cause mortality rate, researchers calculate *YLL* to premature death for each cause of death. Any death from a particular cause is attributed YLLs equal to the highest observed life expectancy minus the age at death. For example, if a man dies of cancer at 65 years of age and his reference life expectancy was 85 years, this would be 20 YLLs due to cancer.[5]

YLL = (highest observed life expectancy for age-of-death cohort) – (age at death)

Nonfatal Outcomes

The key measure of the global burden of nonfatal disease is the *years lived with disability (YLD)*. The YLD requires 2 steps: estimation of the incidence of all disease sequelae (the most detailed outcome modeled, such as mild hearing loss due to otitis media), then multiplying by the disability weight of the condition.

YLD = disease prevalence × disease duration × disability weight

Researchers collect data from government reports, population-based disease registries, hospital discharge data, and many other sources. They then use various tools, such as the DisMod-MR 2.1 (Disease Modeling-Metaregression, a Bayesian metaregression tool developed for GBD), to estimate the prevalence and incidence of all sequelae. Disability weights (described later) are applied to calculate YLDs for conditions ranging from conditions that may last for only a few days (eg, influenza) to those that can last a lifetime (eg, epilepsy).

Disability weights represent the severity of health loss associated with a given health state on a scale from 0 (perfect health) to 1 (disability equal to death).[5] Beginning with the 2010 GBD study, the method of disability weighting is based on large survey data, rather than expert opinion. Large surveys are used to gauge the perceived disability of a condition relative to another condition. Survey participants are asked to choose between descriptions of 2 disabilities (paired comparison) or to express a Time Trade Off for each disability. When applied to multiple socioeconomic and cultural circumstances, such comparisons are an effective and objective way of measuring the *relative* disability of a health state that transcends cultural boundaries. Using surveys of the lay population rather than expert opinion avoids potential bias of the latter but depends on the precise descriptions used. Disability weight descriptions are also intentionally void of any reference to social or economic consequences of disease states. This exclusion can create a problem with accurately assessing the disability related to such conditions as hearing loss and vision loss, whose social and economic impacts go beyond a strict definition of health loss. The differences in survey descriptions and the resulting disability weights for the GBD 2010 and GBD 2013 studies are shown in **Tables 1** and **2**.

Disability-Adjusted Life Year

One DALY can be thought of as one lost year of healthy life. In effect, the DALY combines loss of life with loss of *quality* of life; DALYs are the sum of the YLL and the YLD. The sum of DALYs in a population can be thought of as the gap between the population's present health status and an ideal situation whereby the entire population lives to an advanced age, free of disease.[3,6]

DALY = YLL + YLD

Risk Factor Analysis

GBD risk analysis uses a comparative risk assessment framework to attribute deaths and DALYs to 79 behavioral, environmental and occupational, and metabolic risks. Researchers pool data from various sources, including censuses, surveys, and satellites, to estimate relative risk and exposure. Comparisons of exposure across risks are facilitated through a metric called the summary exposure value (SEV), derived from the combined prevalence of each severity of a risk.[6] Some exposures (eg, smoking) are modeled as categorical risks, whereas others (eg, high systolic blood pressure) are continuous, motivating the SEV approach. GBD 2015 included 388 risk-outcome pairs that satisfied the World Cancer Research Fund–defined criteria for convincing or probable evidence. For each risk-outcome pair, GBD estimates the attributable burden using a counterfactual scenario of the theoretic minimum risk level.

OTHER IMPORTANT GLOBAL BURDEN OF DISEASE METHODS AND CONCEPTS
Impairment Envelope

For certain conditions, health loss is caused by various different diseases; there are better data for the overall impairment than for the impairment due to each cause. GBD models 9 such impairments: anemia, epilepsy, hearing loss, heart failure, intellectual disability, infertility, vision loss, Guillain-Barré syndrome, and pelvic inflammatory disease. For example, there are more data collected on the total prevalence of hearing loss than the prevalence of hearing loss due to meningitis. The impairment strategy is analogous to the cause of death approach (in which

Table 1
Hearing loss disability weights

	Descriptions for the GBD Study 2010	Disability Weights GBD Study 2010	Descriptions for the GBD Study 2013/2015	Disability Weight GBD Study 2015
Hearing loss, mild (20–34 dB)	Has difficulty following a conversation in a noisy environment but no other hearing problems	0.005 (0.002–0.012)	Has great difficulty hearing and understanding another person talking in a noisy place (for example, on an urban street)	0.01 (0.004–0.019)
Hearing loss, moderate (35–49 dB)	Has difficulty hearing a normal voice and great difficulty following a conversation in a noisy environment	0.023 (0.013–0.038)	Is unable to hear and understand another person talking in a noisy place (for example, on an urban street) and has difficulty hearing another person talking even in a quiet place or on the phone	0.027 (0.019–0.042)
Hearing loss, severe (50–79 dB)	Has great difficulty hearing in any situation or in using a phone	0.032 (0.018–0.051)	Is unable to hear and understand another person talking, even in a quiet place, and unable to take part in a phone conversation; emotional impact at times (for example, worry or depression) caused by difficulties with communication and relating to others	0.158 (0.105–0.227)
Hearing loss, profound (80–94 dB)	Always has great difficulty hearing in any situation and is not able to use a phone	0.031 (0.018–0.049)	Is unable to hear and understand another person talking, even in a quiet place, is unable to take part in a phone conversation, and has great difficulty hearing anything in any other situation; worry, depression, and loneliness often caused by difficulties with communicating and relating to others	0.204 (0.134–0.288)

(continued on next page)

Table 1 (continued)				
	Descriptions for the GBD Study 2010	**Disability Weights GBD Study 2010**	**Descriptions for the GBD Study 2013/2015**	**Disability Weight GBD Study 2015**
Hearing loss, complete (95 dB or higher)	Cannot hear at all, even loud sounds	0.033 (0.020–0.052)	Cannot hear at all in any situation, including even the loudest sounds, and cannot communicate verbally or use a phone; worry, depression, or loneliness often caused by difficulties with communicating and relating to others	0.215 (0.144–0.307)

all causes of death must sum to the mortality envelope). GBD estimates the prevalence of each impairment (which the authors refer to herein as the envelope) and ensures that the sum of cause-specific impairment equals the envelope. For some impairments, including hearing, the envelope is estimated for each severity (eg, prevalence of mild hearing loss). The process of developing the hearing loss envelope is outlined in **Fig. 2**.

Cause Hierarchy

The GBD cause list is designed to include the diseases, injuries, and sequelae that are most relevant for public health policy making. The cause list is organized in a hierarchical structure so that different levels of aggregation are included. The cause list is mutually exclusive and collectively exhaustive at every level of aggregation; causes not individually specified are captured in residual categories.[7] There are 3 cause groups within level 1: communicable, maternal, neonatal, and nutritional diseases (group 1 diseases); noncommunicable diseases (group 2); and injuries (group 3). At level 2 of the hierarchy these groups are subdivided into 21 cause groupings (eg, neonatal disorders, neurologic disorders, and transport injuries). Levels 3 and 4 contain the finest level of detail for causes captured in GBD 2015. In the GBD 2015 study, the following causes of hearing loss were modeled at level 4: congenital, meningitis, otitis, and age-related and other.[8] Laryngeal, lip and oral cavity, nasopharyngeal, and other pharyngeal cancers are listed in the cause hierarchy at level 3. Otitis media is also listed in the cause hierarchy at level 3, but hearing loss as a sequela of otitis media is listed at level 4. Levels 5 and 6 are composed of the most detailed consequences estimated, sequelae. Sequelae are mutually exclusive consequences of diseases and injuries, and each is connected to a specific cause. For example, acute otitis media and mild hearing loss due to chronic otitis media are both sequelae of otitis media.

Sequelae of diseases and injuries are organized at levels 5 and 6 of the hierarchy. In GBD, sequelae are defined as distinct, mutually exclusive categories of health consequences. For example, both neuropathy and diabetic retinopathy are sequelae of diabetes, whereas, stroke and ischemic heart disease are not,

Table 2
Hearing loss with tinnitus disability weights

	Descriptions for the GBD Study 2010	Disability Weights GBD Study 2010	Descriptions for the GBD Study 2013/2015	Disability Weight GBD Study 2015
Hearing loss, mild, with ringing	Has great difficulty following a conversation in a noisy environment and has ringing in the ears for more than 5 min, almost every day	0.038 (0.024–0.058)	Has great difficulty hearing and understanding another person talking in a noisy place (for example, on an urban street) and sometimes has annoying ringing in the ears	0.021 (0.012–0.036)
Hearing loss, moderate, with ringing	Has difficulty hearing a normal voice or using a phone, has great difficulty following a conversation in a noisy environment, and has ringing in the ears for more than 5 min, almost every day	0.058 (0.037–0.085)	Is unable to hear and understand another person talking in a noisy place (for example, on an urban street), has difficulty hearing another person talking even in a quiet place or on the phone, and has annoying ringing in the ear for 5 min at a time, almost every day	0.074 (0.049–0.107)
Hearing loss, severe, with ringing	Has great difficulty hearing in any situation or in using a phone and has ringing in the ears for more than 5 min, almost every day	0.065 (0.041–0.094)	Is unable to hear and understand another person talking, even in a quiet place, is unable to take part in a phone conversation, and has annoying ringing in the ear for more than 5 min at a time, almost every day; emotional impact at times (for example, worry or depression) caused by difficulties with communication and relating to others	0.261 (0.175–0.36)

(continued on next page)

Table 2
(continued)

	Descriptions for the GBD Study 2010	Disability Weights GBD Study 2010	Descriptions for the GBD Study 2013/2015	Disability Weight GBD Study 2015
Hearing loss, profound, with ringing	Always has great difficulty hearing in any situation, cannot use a phone, and has ringing in the ears for more than 5 min, almost every day	0.088 (0.058–0.127)	Is unable to hear and understand another person talking, even in a quiet place, is unable to take part in a phone conversation, has great difficulty hearing anything in any other situation, and has annoying ringing in the ear for more than 5 min at a time, several times a day; worry, depression, and loneliness often caused by difficulties with communicating and relating to others	0.277 (0.182–0.387)
Hearing loss, complete, with ringing	Cannot hear at all, even loud sounds, cannot use a phone, and has ringing in the ears for more than 5 min, almost every day	0.092 (0.061–0.134)	Cannot hear at all in any situation, including even the loudest sounds, and cannot communicate verbally or use a phone, and has very annoying ringing in the ears for more than half of the day; worry, depression, or loneliness often caused by difficulties with communicating and relating to others	0.316 (0.212–0.435)

as these consequences cannot be categorically ascribed to diabetes despite good evidence for increased risk of these outcomes. Because sequelae estimates in GBD are mutually exclusive and collectively exhaustive, the YLD estimates at each level of the hierarchy sum to the total of the level above. In contrast, prevalence estimates are not additive, as individuals may have more than one sequela or disease.

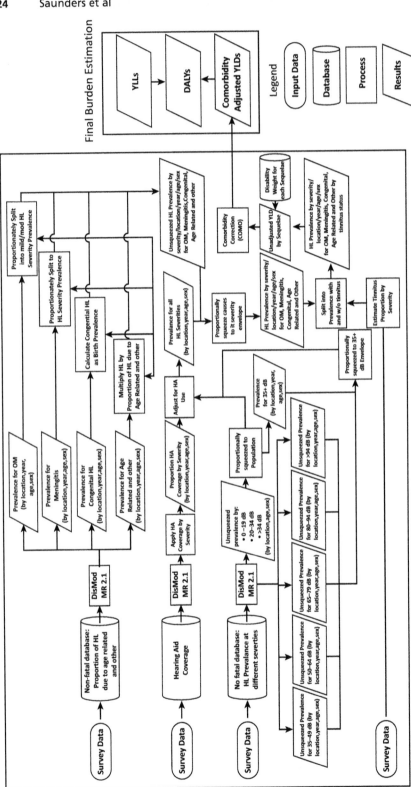

Fig. 2. Flowchart for Deriving non-fatal disability burden in Years Lived with Disease for hearing loss, including the process of developing the impairment envelope. Note that prevalence estimates are segregated according to severity ("unsqueezed") and re-aggregated ("squeezed") to a final estimate. HL, hearing Loss; HA, hearing aid. (*Adapted from* GBD 2016 Disease and Injury Incidence and Prevalence Collaborators. Global, regional, and national incidence, prevalence, and years lived with disability for 328 diseases and injuries for 195 countries, 1990–2016: a systematic analysis for the Global Burden of Disease Study 2016. Lancet 2017;390:1211–59; with permission.)

Geographic, Age, and Sex Definitions

There are 20 age groupings in the 2015 GBD; also, estimates are reported by sex and for both sexes combined.[6,8] GBD 2015 modeled the following detailed age groups: early neonatal (0–6 days), late neonatal (7–27 days), postneonatal (28–364 days), 1 to 4 years, and the 5-year age group until the 80-years + age group. For GBD 2016, the 80-years + age group is replaced with 80 to 84, 85 to 89, and estimate 5-year age groups up to 95+. IHME aggregates estimates to various age groups of interest, including less than 5 years, 5 to 14, 15 to 49, all ages, and age standardized. GBD reports for males, females, and both sexes combined. The 21 geographic regions (including 195 countries) of the GBD 2015 study were created based on epidemiologic similarity and geographic proximity. For some types of analysis in the GBD, 7 super-regions have been established. **Fig. 3** shows the 7 GBD super-regions and 21 regions within.[5]

Statistical Methods and Terms

Some important statistical terms/techniques are defined in the glossary of terms (**Table 3**). The GBD includes uncertainty intervals that reflect a range of values that are likely to include the correct estimate of health loss for a given cause. Larger uncertainty intervals can result from limited data availability, small studies, and conflicting data, whereas smaller uncertainty intervals can result from extensive data availability, large studies, and data that are consistent across sources.[9] GBD propagates uncertainty through multistep analytical processes by repeating calculations over 1000 draws, using distributions of plausible values rather than mean estimates. This task is computationally intensive given the large number of diseases and injuries and their sequelae.[10]

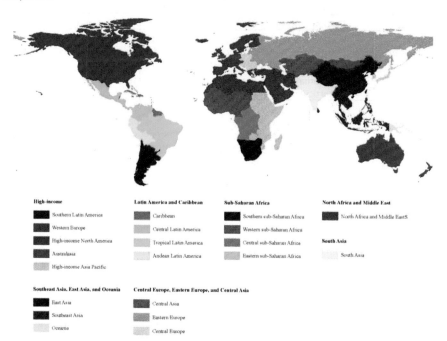

Fig. 3. GBD geographic regions. (*Courtesy of* Institute of Health Metrics and Evaluation, Seattle (WA); with permission.)

Table 3
Glossary of terms

Term	Definition
DALY	The YLL due to premature mortality in the population and the YLD for people living with the health condition or its consequences
YLD	An abbreviation for years lived with disability, which can also be described as years lived in less than ideal health
YLL	Calculated by subtracting the age at death from the longest possible life expectancy for a person at that age
Disability weights	Represent the severity of health loss associated with a given health state on a scale from 0 (perfect health) to 1 (disability equal to death)
Life expectancy	A measure that reflects the overall mortality level of a population
HALE	The average number of years that a person can expect to live in full health by taking into account years lived in less than full health due to disease and/or injury (YLDs) and years lost due to premature mortality (YLLs) in a single measure of average population health for individual countries
Mortality envelopes	An overall estimate of number of deaths by given demographics, such as age, sex, and/or cause
Health states	Groupings of sequelae that reflect key differences in symptoms and functioning; different health states assigned different disability weight valuations
Age-standardization	A statistical technique used to compare populations with different age structures, in which the characteristics of the populations are statistically transformed to match those of a reference population
SEV	A measure of a population's exposure to a risk factor that takes into account the extent of exposure (risk level) and the severity of that risk's contribution to disease burden
Sequelae	Consequences that are directly attributable to diseases and injuries
Age standardization	A statistical technique to compare populations with different age structures, in which the characteristics of the populations are statistically transformed to match those of a reference population
Attributable burden	An estimate of the share of a burden of disease that occurs due to a particular risk factor
SDI	A summary measure expressed on a scale of 0–1 intended to identify where countries or regions are on the spectrum of development; is a composite average of the rankings of the incomes per capita, average educational attainment, and fertility rates of all areas in the GBD study
1000 Draws	A method of determining uncertainty intervals through repeated sampling of the GBD database
DisMod-MR 2.1	Disease modeling-meta-regression, a Bayesian meta-regression tool developed for GBD

Abbreviations: HALE, healthy life expectancy; SDI, Sociodemographic Index.

Data from Institute for Health Metrics and Evaluation (IHME). Rethinking development and health: findings from the Global Burden of Disease study. Seattle (WA): IHME; 2016. Available at: http://www.healthdata.org/sites/default/files/files/policy_report/GBD/2016/IHME_GBD2015_report.pdf; and Institute for Health Metrics and Evaluation (IHME). Frequently asked questions. Seattle (WA): University of Washington; 2018. Available at: http://www.healthdata.org/gbd/faq.

Process and Collaborator Input

The GBD Collaborator Network engages individual collaborators with expertise on all-cause mortality; specific diseases, injuries, risk factors, and impairments; and country-specific epidemiology. GBD's 1600 collaborators from 120 countries include researchers, scientists, university professors, policymakers, government health offi-cials, staff of nongovernmental organizations, students, and people implementing public health programs.[1] GBD collaborators are invited to collaborate in the following ways (see also http://www.healthdata.org/gbd/call-for-collaborators):

- Assess data sources being used and suggest new data sources, including those from literature, surveys, administrative data, hospital data, registries, and other related sources
- Provide data of their own to integrate into the analyses
- Critique results from the estimation
- Suggest new causes, risk factors, and risk-outcome pairs
- Give feedback on covariates and modeling approaches
- Provide critique and feedback on articles
- Contribute to articles and participate as investigators
- Carry out related analyses using GBD data
- Disseminate results at conferences, workshops, and other avenues of interest
- Participate in media outreach
- Refer colleagues as collaborators
- Jointly pursue funding opportunities of mutual interest
- Take part in select training opportunities and be alerted of opportunities to expand the impact of the GBD through conferences, networks, and calls for abstracts

SPECIFIC OTOLARYNGOLOGY DISEASES IN THE GLOBAL BURDEN OF DISEASE
Hearing Loss

Globally, hearing loss is the fourth most common chronic disease by prevalence in the GBD 2015 study (preceded by dental caries, headaches, and iron deficiency anemia).[11] The GBD prevalence of any hearing loss (>20 dB) is estimated at 1.2 billion, which is 28% more than the 2005 estimate. There has been a steady increase in estimates for age-related and other hearing loss with a 26.4% increase in YLDs from 2005 and a total YLD of 40.59 million in 2015 (**Fig. 4**). Hearing loss contributes 5.1% of the global YLDs for all causes, slightly higher than the YLDs due to diabetes.[12] These increases arise in large part from the globally aging population and overall population growth. GBD decomposition analyses suggest that the aging world population contributes roughly half of the increases in sense organ disease since 2005. As hearing loss is not a fatal disease, the DALY estimates are the same as the YLD (40.59 million). Hearing loss constitutes 1.64% of the total DALYs in the world, a comparable global health burden to tuberculosis, and is ranked 15th in global DALY contribution (see **Fig. 1**).

Although there have been some improvements in epidemiologic data for hearing loss, there are still large gaps; high-quality, international data are limited. The GBD reports that data are only available for hearing loss from 16.5% of all geographic areas. In 2015, Ped-erson and colleagues[13] reviewed the Cochrane database for otolaryngologic diseases with the GBD data on how much these diseases impact global health. They concluded that hearing loss is the most underrepresented condition of otolaryngologic diseases.

Overall, hearing loss is associated with male sex and age as well as low- and middle-income regions.[14] In the GBD 2015 study, hearing loss is estimated for 3 dis-eases states: otitis media, meningitis, and congenital disorders. Higher rates of hear-ing loss in lower-income areas may be secondary to increased rates of these conditions. All other hearing loss cases (more than 90% of the hearing loss preva-lence) are included in the age-related and other category. Most clinicians would agree that this is a rather broad grouping; but unfortunately data on hearing loss cause are

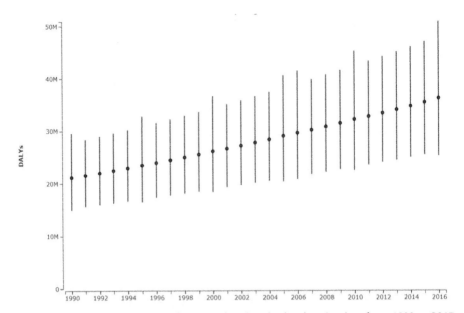

Fig. 4. GBD prevalence estimates for age-related and other hearing loss from 1990 to 2015 in millions (M). (*Data from* Institute for Health Metrics and Evaluation (IHME). GBD compare. Seattle (WA): IHME, University of Washington; 2018. Available at: http://vizhub.healthdata. org/gbd-compare.)

lacking, especially in low-resource countries where prevalence is highest. Some other diseases within the GBD cause hierarchy that are known to cause hearing loss include human immunodeficiency virus, tuberculosis, rubella, and Down syndrome.[15–21] Occupational noise exposure has been analyzed as a risk factor for age-related and other hearing loss, with an estimated contribution of 26.79% of the overall DALYs.

In children, hearing loss from unspecified causes are also included in the age-related and other hearing loss category. All of the specified causes with hearing loss sequelae that are recognized by the GBD (ie, meningitis, congenital and otitis media) typically affected children more than adults. The disability from these causes is more difficult to isolate with current reporting practices. In a specific study of children and adolescents (0–19 years of age), the prevalence of hearing loss that is not elsewhere classified (age related and other) was estimated to be 53.3 million worldwide (a 5.7% increase from the 2005 report). The prevalence and YLD estimates for all causes of hearing loss combined (including sequelae of otitis media, all forms of meningitis, and congenital anomalies) in this report were reported to be 109.3 million and 6.48 million, respectively (**Table 4**). By comparison, the same estimates for all causes of vision loss are 113.8 million and 3.28 million.

One of the most difficult aspects of measuring the global burden due to hearing loss is the accurate estimation of the disability of the condition. Disability weight surveys struggle to account for the secondary effect of severe hearing loss on language development and communication as well as the significant effect of the age of onset on this aspect of the condition. Clinicians working in this field recognize that the disability caused by the hearing loss varies greatly, with childhood hearing loss or profound hearing loss having a much greater impact. Impaired language skills can also lead to reduced education and economic productivity; however, disability weight surveys specifically exclude references to such educational and economic consequences as

Table 4
Child and adolescent (0–19 y) hearing loss estimates for prevalence and years of life lost

Hearing Loss Cause	2015 Prevalence	Prevalence Change from 2005 (%)	2015 YLDs	YLD Change from 2005 (%)
Age-related and other	53,295,156	+5.7	3,781,468	+4.5
Otitis media	43,457,019	+1.1	1,737,171	−0.4
Congenital	11,941,073	+4.7	918,444	+2.2
Pneumococcal meningitis	298,152	+24.6	23,603	+22.6
Other meningitis	102,560	+18.4	8126	+17.2
Haemophilus influenza type B meningitis	103,281	−24.8	8183	−26.9
Meningococcal meningitis	70,958	+19.1	5768	+16.9
All causes	109,268,199	+3.7	6,482,765	+2.8

From Kassebaum N. Child and adolescent health from 1990 to 2015: findings from the global burden of diseases, injuries, and risk factors 2015 study. JAMA Pediatr 2017;171(6):573–92; with permission.

noted earlier. The current GBD disability weight descriptions do, however, include the possible mental health consequences (depression and loneliness) of severe to complete hearing loss. The addition of this terminology and stronger, more specific wording resulted in a significant revision of the hearing loss disability weights in the GBD 2013 study (see **Table 1**). The GBD hearing loss disability weights do not factor in the increased disability for the onset of severe hearing loss before language development. In contrast, hearing loss with tinnitus does result in a slightly higher disability weight (see **Table 2**). Before the revised disability weights for hearing loss in the GBD 2013 studies, mild hearing loss with tinnitus resulted in a higher disability weight than complete hearing loss. This revision is an excellent example of the GBD responsiveness to feedback from collaborators and experts.[22]

In GBD methodology, the use of hearing aids lowers the estimated disability weights by one level. For example, a person with severe hearing loss using a hearing aid would be estimated to have the same disability as a person with moderate hearing loss. This assumption arises from a lack of data on hearing aid effectiveness and does not address the range of quality of health care and technology available. Although most cases of hearing loss can be treated effectively with hearing aids, most people with a hearing impairment live in low-resource countries with very poor access to hearing aids. The GBD estimates the proportion of people with a hearing impairment who use hearing aids in each country. There are reasonable data on the use of hearing aids in higher-income countries but very little data on the availability of this technology in low- or middle-income countries. Hearing aid coverage is estimated to be relatively flat from 1990 to 2015, but the model predicts increasing hearing aid coverage with age and with female sex (**Fig. 5**). The availability and potential impact of cochlear implants on the burden of profound or complete hearing loss is even less clear. Most agree this technology is only available to a very small fraction (<1%) of potential candidates in low-resource populations.

Otitis Media

Otitis media is another common otolaryngologic condition that contributes to the global burden of disease.[11,23] In the 2015 rankings, it is the third most common short-term disease with an incidence of 471 million. The prevalence for both chronic

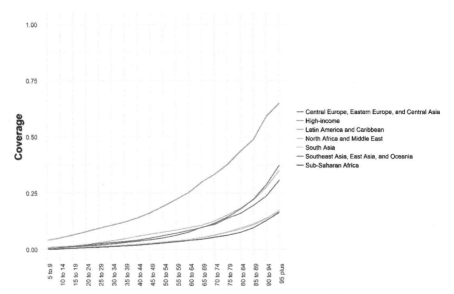

Fig. 5. Estimated hearing aid coverage for GBD super-regions (2016 data). Percentage of individuals with hearing loss (>20 dB) who use hearing aids. (*Data from* Global Burden of Disease Study 2016. Global Burden of Disease Study 2016 (GBD 2016) results. Seattle (WA): Institute for Health Metrics and Evaluation (IHME); 2017.)

and acute otitis media is estimated to be 112 million. The prevalence and global impact slightly declined from the 2005 report, with a current DALY estimated at 3.50 million, comprising only 0.14% of the world DALY total in spite of the high prevalence. This relatively low DALY estimate is due in part to the short-term nature of the acute otitis media and a low disability weight. Both acute otitis media and severe infectious complications of otitis media are allotted a disability weight of 0.013. The current disability weights associated with otitis media consider mainly ear pain and most (97%) chronic otitis media is considered asymptomatic. A separate report on the child and adolescent global burden of disease cites a prevalence of 43.5 million and 1.7 million YLDs for otitis media in children 0 to 19 years of age.[24]

Cleft Lip and Palate

Cleft lip and palate contribute a relatively small amount to global disease burden but are found to be disproportionally represented in the Cochrane Database of Systematic Reviews based on this minor contribution to total DALYs.[13] Children born with cleft lip and palate can experience feeding difficulties, speech delays, and emotional trauma from the disfiguring condition. These factors are taken into account when calculating the disability associated with the disease.[7] The prevalence in 2015 was 6.88 million (0.96 million DALYs), a 44.8% decrease from the 2005.

Head and Neck Cancer

Head and neck cancers included in the cause hierarchy include lip, oral, nasopharyngeal, pharyngeal, laryngeal, esophageal, and thyroid cancer. Salivary gland cancers are included under *other neoplasms*. Overall head and neck cancer has an increased burden of disease when compared with the 2005 impact (**Table 5**). All head and neck cancers have increased in prevalence over the past decade along with the associated

Table 5 Global Burden of Disease 2015 head and neck cancer disability-adjusted life years					
Cancer	2015 Prevalence	Prevalence Change from 2005 (%)	2015 YLDs	DALYs	DALY Change from 2005 (%)
Lip and oral	2425.1	38.6	209.1	3780.1	28.0
Nasopharynx	732.7	18.0	69.7	1911.7	5.9
Pharynx	945.5	32.7	79.5	1715.7	20.8
Larynx	1412.6	26.2	147.3	2608.5	10.3
Thyroid	3166.5	101.1	190.0	846.3	30.3
Esophageal	746	19.6	128.6	9854.4	−7.6

All numbers reported in thousands.
Data from Institute for Health Metrics and Evaluation. Protocol for the global burden of disease, injuries, and risk factors study (GBD) v.2. Seattle (WA): IHME; 2015; and Murray CJ, Lopez AD, Jamison DT. The global burden of disease in 1990: summary results, sensitivity analysis and future directions. Bull World Health Organ 1994;72(3):495–509.

DALYs. However, the percentage of DALYs from esophageal cancer has decreased and age-standardized rates have decreased for all head and neck cancers except thyroid and oral (**Fig. 6**). Collectively, all of these cancers still contribute less than 1% of global DALYs, with the largest contribution from esophageal cancer (0.4%).[12] Esophageal cancer accounts for almost 50% of the DALYs from head and neck cancer and is underrepresented in the literature based on its contribution to the burden of disease.[13] Recent efforts by the GBD have sought to determine the percent of head and neck cancer health burden that is directly attributable to tobacco and alcohol abuse. The attributable risks for smoking for laryngeal, lip and oral cavity, and nasopharyngeal cancers are 61.8%, 40.9%, and 33.6% of the total DALYs, respectively.

Trauma

One of the important contributions of the GBD is the recognition of the impact of trauma on the overall burden of disease in the world. This recognition has led to a growing

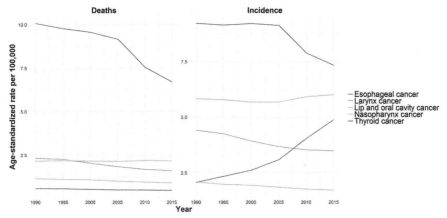

Fig. 6. Head and neck cancer trends: incidence and DALYs. (*Data from* Global Burden of Disease Study 2016. Global Burden of Disease Study 2016 (GBD 2016) Results. Seattle (WA): Institute for Health Metrics and Evaluation (IHME); 2017.)

recognition of the importance of both road safety as a critical aspect of global health and the need for adequate surgical services to treat trauma victims in low-resource areas. Unfortunately, head and neck injuries from trauma are difficult to isolate. Countries generally report trauma by the nature of the injury or by the cause of injury, but very few report both. Although trauma patients often have multiple injuries, the GBD estimates the trauma burden according to the nature (site) of the injury for only the most severe injury. Facial trauma is commonly associated with neurologic injuries (assigned higher importance). The GBD is currently classifying more detailed information about the site of injury in a series of N-codes (nature of injury). These codes include injuries relevant to otolaryngology, including facial and skull fractures, as well as foreign bodies of the ear and airway burns. Eventually these codes will be linked to external causes of injuries or E-codes (external cause of injury, eg, motor vehicle accident) and estimated specific DALY allotments estimated for each component of the trauma. Such data will be helpful in determining resource allocation and training needs.

Oral Disorders

With an estimated prevalence of 3.53 billion (increased from 3.08 billion in 2005) resulting in 16.96 million DALYs, oral disorders have the highest prevalence of any GBD cause. Consequently, they contribute significant demands on the health system despite low disability weights. Oral disorders include dental contributions, such as deciduous caries, permanent caries, periodontal diseases, edentulism, and severe tooth loss. In addition, otolaryngology-related diseases in the other oral disorders category encompasses tongue, jaw, and other oral malformations.[12]

FUTURE DIRECTIONS AND POTENTIAL ROLE OF OTOLARYNGOLOGISTS

The GBD project is a critically important advancement that provides an objective assessment of global health and epidemiologic trends. This work has great potential to improve otolaryngology health care globally and prevent many of the diseases otolaryngologists treat. With an improved understanding of the burden of disease in the world, health policy makers are already beginning to realize the importance of noncommunicable diseases and surgical care.

The prominent prevalence and disability of hearing loss in the GBD analysis emphasizes the need to support training programs and services in audiology and otologic surgery. The GBD analysis clearly demonstrates the effect of an aging population on hearing loss. Although low resources often limit the capacity to expand programs for hearing loss, the objective estimates from the GBD underscores their importance.

Risk factor analysis points to needed improvements in road safety and reduced tobacco use, with respective potential impacts on facial trauma and head and neck cancer. Longitudinal data from GBD reveals interesting trends in the incidence of most head and neck cancers, especially esophageal cancer. The cause and significance of this trend is unclear, but only through detailed analysis would such trends become evident.

In spite of these observations, efforts to improve global otolaryngology health care are limited by the available data. More effort is needed to gather high-quality epidemiologic data on otolaryngology diseases including the following:

- The prevalence of these diseases, especially in low-resource areas of the world (eg, population surveys for adult hearing loss, newborn screening data for child hearing loss, and disease registries for cancers).
- The degree of disability caused by these diseases, such as hearing loss and otitis media (eg, the psychological effects of untreated severe hearing loss)

- The specific cause and severity of hearing loss in low-resource areas and the utilization of hearing technology (eg, hearing aids) in these areas
- The prevalence of hearing loss as sequelae of other diseases in the GBD cause hierarchy (eg, tuberculosis and rubella)
- Additional risk factor contribution (exposure) to otolaryngologic diseases (eg, occupational noise exposure for hearing loss)

Understanding the cause and risk factors associated with these diseases is the first step toward primary prevention. Improved DALY and YLD estimates can contribute to improved prevention strategies. Gathering high-quality data on these topics will require the commitment of otolaryngologists and researchers around the world. In return, the information gained from this effort will aid in convincing policymakers and clinicians to make informed decisions about health care priorities. Ultimately, the application of this knowledge may help to reduce the burden of otolaryngologic diseases and improve otolaryngology health care globally.

ACKNOWLEDGMENTS

The authors wish to thank the following people at the University of Washington Institute for Health Metrics and Evaluation for their invaluable support in the preparation of this article: Pauline Kim, Kate Muller, Joan Williams, and Helen E. Olsen.

REFERENCES

1. Institute for Health Metrics and Evaluation (IHME). Protocol for the global burden of diseases, injuries, and risk factors study (GBD). Version 2.0. Seattle (WA): IHME; 2015. Available at: http://www.healthdata.org/sites/default/files/files/Projects/GBD/GBD_Protocol.pdf. Accessed March 3, 2018.
2. Murray CJ, Lopez AD, Jamison DT. The global burden of disease in 1990: summary results, sensitivity analysis and future directions. Bull World Health Organ 1994;72(3):495–509.
3. Institute for Health Metrics and Evaluation (IHME). Rethinking development and health: findings of the global burden of disease study. Seattle (WA): IHME; 2016. Available at: http://www.healthdata.org/sites/default/files/files/policy_report/GBD/2016/IHME_GBD2015_report.pdf. Accessed March 3, 2018.
4. Lozano R, Naghavi M, Foreman K, et al, GBD 2010 Disease and Injury Incidence and Prevalence Collaborators. Global and regional mortality from 235 causes of death for 20 age groups in 1990 and 2010: a systematic analysis for the Global Burden of Disease Study 2010. Lancet 2012;380(9859):2095–128. Available at: http://thelancet.com/journals/lancet/article/PIIS0140-6736(12)61728-0/fulltext. Accessed March 3, 2018.
5. Institute for Health Metrics and Evaluation (IHME). Frequently asked questions. Available at: http://www.healthdata.org/gbd/faq. Accessed March 3, 2018.
6. GBD 2015 Risk Factors Collaborators. Global, regional, and national comparative risk assessment of 79 behavioural, environmental and occupational, and metabolic risks or clusters of risks, 1990–2015: a systematic analysis for the Global Burden of Disease Study 2015. Lancet 2016;388(10053):1659–724. Available at: http://thelancet.com/journals/lancet/article/PIIS0140-6736(16)31679-8/fulltext. Accessed March 3, 2018.
7. Institute of Health Metrics and Evaluation Website: GBD Cause List. Available at: http://www.healthdata.org/sites/default/files/files/Projects/GBD/GBDcause_list.pdf. Accessed March 3, 2018.

8. Institute of Health Metrics and Evaluation Website: GBD Cause List. Available at: http://www.healthdata.org/sites/default/files/files/Projects/GBD/GBDAges.pdf. Accessed March 3, 2018.

9. Institute of Health Metrics and Evaluation Website: terms defined. Available at: http://www.healthdata.org/terms-defined. Accessed March 3, 2018.

10. Murray CJ, Ezzati M, Flaxman AD, et al. Supplement to: GBD 2010: design, definitions, and metrics. Lancet 2012;380(9859):2063–6. Available at: http://www.thelancet.com/cms/attachment/2017336178/2037711222/mmc1.pd. Accessed March 3, 2018.

11. GBD 2015 Disease and Injury Incidence and Prevalence Collaborators. Global, regional, and national incidence, prevalence, and years lived with disability for 310 diseases and injuries, 1990–2015: a systematic analysis for the Global Burden of Disease Study 2015. Lancet 2016;388(10053):1545–602.

12. GBD 2015 DALYs and HALE Collaborators. Global, regional, and national disability-adjusted life-years (DALYs) for 315 diseases and injuries and healthy life expectancy (HALE), 1990–2015: a systematic analysis for the global burden of disease study 2015. Lancet 2016;388(10053):1603–58.

13. Pederson H, Okland T, Boyers LN, et al. Identifying otolaryngology systematic review research gaps: comparing global burden of disease 2010 results with Cochrane database of systematic review. JAMA Otolaryngol Head Neck Surg 2015;141(1):67–72.

14. Stevens G, Flaxman S, Brunskill E, et al. Global burden of disease hearing loss expert group global and regional hearing impairment prevalence: an analysis of 42 studies in 29 countries. Eur J Public Health 2013;23(1):146–52.

15. Maro II, Moshi N, Clavier OH, et al. Auditory impairments in HIV-infected individuals in Tanzania. Ear Hear 2014;35(3):306–17.

16. Seddon JA, Thee S, Jacobs K, et al. Hearing loss in children treated for multidrug-resistant tuberculosis. J Infect 2013;66(4):320–9.

17. Lasisi OA, Ayodele JK, Ijaduola GT. Challenges in management of childhood sensorineural hearing loss in sub-Saharan Africa, Nigeria. Int J Pediatr Otorhinolaryngol 2006;70(4):625–9.

18. Thompson KM, Simons EA, Badizadegan K, et al. Characterization of the risks of adverse outcomes following rubella infection in pregnancy. Risk Anal 2016;36(7):1315–31.

19. Caroça C, Vicente V, Campelo P, et al. Rubella in sub-Saharan Africa and sensorineural hearing loss: a case control study. BMC Public Health 2017;17(1):146.

20. Roisen NJ, Wolters C, Nicol T, et al. Hearing loss in children with Down syndrome. J Pediatr 1993;123(1):S9–12.

21. McPherson B, Lai SP, Leung KK, et al. Hearing loss in Chinese school children with Down syndrome. Int J Pediatr Otorhinolaryngol 2007;71(12):1905–15.

22. Salomon JA, Haagsma JA, Davis A, et al. Disability weights for the global burden of disease 2013 study. Lancet Glob Health 2015;3(11):e712–23.

23. Monasta L, Ronfani L, Marchetti F, et al. Burden of disease caused by otitis media: systematic review and global estimates. PLoS One 2012;7(4):e36226.

24. Kassebaum N, Arora M, Barber RM, et al. Child and adolescent health from 1990 to 2015. JAMA Pediatr 2017;123(1):199–206.

World Health Organization and Its Initiative for Ear and Hearing Care

Shelly Chadha, MBBS, MSurg (ENT), PhD (Public Health)*,
Alarcos Cieza, MSc (Psychology), PhD (Medical Psychology)

KEYWORDS

- Global hearing • Hearing loss • Ear and hearing care • Prevention of deafness
- Hearing loss prevention • World hearing day • World Health Association resolution

KEY POINTS

- The World Health Organization (WHO) is the United Nations' specialized agency in the field of health.
- WHO addresses ear and hearing problems through its program for prevention of deafness and hearing loss.
- The World Health Assembly recently adopted a resolution highlighting the need for global and national action to deal with hearing loss.
- Based on this resolution, WHO has identified 4 key strategic work areas for the coming 5 years.
- WHO calls upon all stakeholders, including ear and hearing care professionals, to come together in order to drive global action for hearing loss.

INTRODUCTION

As the global leader in the field of public health, the World Health Organization (WHO) addresses health issues that are prioritized by its Member States[a]. These include a diverse variety of areas addressing infections such as malaria, tuberculosis, polio, and acquired immunodeficiency syndrome (AIDS); reducing mortality and morbidity due to conditions such as heart disease, diabetes and cancer; promoting road safety, violence prevention; and many more areas.[1] The issues that are included in WHO's program of work are typically those that have been highlighted as public health issues

---

Disclosure: The authors have nothing to disclose.
WHO Department for Management of NCDs, Disability, Violence and Injury Prevention, World Health Organization, Avenue Appia 20, Geneva 1211, Switzerland
* Corresponding author.
E-mail address: chadhas@who.int

[a] Member State refers to the 194 countries that are members of the United Nations system.

Otolaryngol Clin N Am 51 (2018) 535–542
https://doi.org/10.1016/j.otc.2018.01.002
0030-6665/18/© 2018 Elsevier Inc. All rights reserved.

of global importance based on their prevalence, impact, and prioritization by governments and civil society groups.

Relevant to the field of otolaryngology, hearing loss has been prioritized in consequence of its rising prevalence and the importance of hearing as a contributor toward optimal health in all ages. WHO initiated a program for prevention of deafness and hearing loss in the late 1990s to address hearing loss and ear diseases that lead to it. This program has gradually evolved over the last 20 years and recently been strengthened by a newly adopted World Health Assembly resolution. The program is driving a multistakeholder global effort to make ear and hearing care accessible for all people across different regions and income settings. This article summarizes the role that WHO plays in global health, while outlining specifically its strategies for addressing ear problems and hearing loss. It also looks at the importance of coordinated multi-stakeholder global action and makes suggestions about how all professionals can contribute toward this effort.

THE WORLD HEALTH ORGANIZATION

WHO was established in the aftermath of World War II as the United Nations' specialized agency in the field of health.[1] As the world's directing and coordinating authority on international health, WHO aims to build a better, healthier future for people all over the world. To achieve the sustainable development goal for health: *Ensure healthy lives and promote well-being,* WHO has identified 6 priority areas for action. These are

- Advancing universal health coverage: enabling countries to sustain or expand access to all needed health services and financial protection, and promoting universal health coverage
- Achieving health-related development goals: addressing unfinished and future challenges relating to maternal and child health; combating HIV, malaria, tuberculosis; and completing the eradication of polio and several neglected tropical diseases
- Addressing the challenge of noncommunicable diseases and mental health, violence, and injuries and disabilities
- Ensuring that all countries can detect and respond to acute public health threats under the international health regulations
- Increasing access to quality, safe, efficacious, and affordable medical products (medicines, vaccines, diagnostics, and other health technologies)
- Addressing the social, economic, and environmental determinants of health as a means to promote health outcomes and reduce health inequalities within and between countries

WHO works in close collaboration with the ministries of health of its 194 member states, that is, countries that are part of the United Nations. The headquarters of WHO works closely with its 6 regional offices and over 150 country offices alongside the national governments to ensure the implementation of its ambitious agenda.

The ministries of health of national governments are a key part of the World Health Assembly, which is the supreme decision-making body in global health and guides WHO's agenda and work. Besides governments, WHO partners with many professional, nongovernmental, and civil society organizations and draws upon the knowledge and resources of a large body of experts to guide it in the development of evidence-based policies and recommendations.

HEARING LOSS: CAUSE FOR CONCERN

In 1995, the World Health Assembly discussed the issue of the rising prevalence of hearing loss across the world and highlighted the need to address this as a public health issue through the primary health care systems of countries. A resolution for prevention of hearing impairment was adopted (WHA 48.9, 1995) that outlined actions for countries and WHO to undertake to address this issue.[2] Over the years that followed this resolution, WHO developed materials, resources, and guidelines to support countries in its implementation.

Despite this, only 32 member states reported setting up national strategies and plans to address ear diseases and hearing loss[3] (**Fig. 1**).

Meanwhile, disabling hearing loss was estimated to now affect over 5% of the world's population and be a leading contributor to morbidity globally (estimated by calculating disability-adjusted life years [DALYs] and years lived with disability [YLDs]).[4,5] A recent report also confirmed that unaddressed hearing loss poses a high financial cost, with an estimated $750 billion being lost annually.[6]

Concern is also raised about the increasing prevalence and impact of hearing loss. In 2015, WHO estimated that over 1 billion young people are at risk of hearing loss because of the way they listen to music.[7] Also, there is a significant demographic shift, with an increasing number of older adults globally, a third of whom are likely to have hearing loss requiring interventions.[8]

SOLUTIONS EXIST

Analyzing the etiology of hearing loss reveals that many of its causes are preventable. As a matter of fact, 60% of hearing loss cases in children are attributed to preventable causes that include ear infections, infectious diseases such as rubella and meningitis, birth-related complications, noise exposure, and ototoxicity.[9] Studies also show that when hearing loss occurs, early intervention programs for timely identification and rehabilitation can mitigate its adverse impact and are cost-effective to implement[6] (**Fig. 2**).

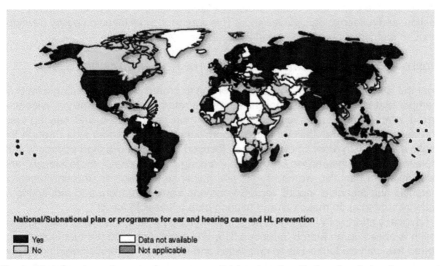

National/Subnational plan or programme for ear and hearing care and HL prevention

■ Yes   ☐ Data not available
☐ No   ▨ Not applicable

Fig. 1. Map showing existence of government-initiated national/subnational plan for ear and hearing care. (*From* Chestnov O, Mendis M, Chadha S, et al. Multicountry assessment of national capacity to provide hearing care. Geneva (Switzerland): World Health Organization (WHO). 2013. Available at: http://www.who.int/pbd/publications/WHOReportHearingCare_Englishweb.pdf. Accessed July 31, 2017; with permission.)

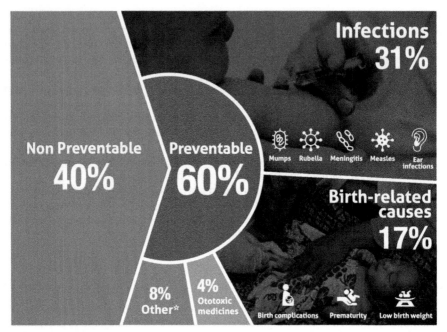

Fig. 2. Distribution of preventable causes of childhood hearing loss. (*From* Krug E, Chadha S, Sminkey L, et al. Childhood hearing loss: strategies for prevention and care. World Health Organization (WHO). 2016. Available at: http://apps.who.int/iris/bitstream/10665/204632/1/9789241510325_eng.pdf?ua=1. Accessed July 31, 2017; with permission.)

What is required is a public health approach toward this subject. Such an approach should include population-based strategies such as health promotion, disease prevention, and epidemiologic surveillance. This approach must focus on policy development, implementation, and monitoring of multi-stakeholder action.

WORLD HEALTH ORGANIZATION ACTIONS IN THE FIELD OF HEARING LOSS

Over the last few years, WHO has been working to promote ear and hearing care in its member states. The term ear and hearing care refers to comprehensive, evidence-based interventions to prevent, identify, and treat ear diseases and hearing loss, and to habilitate or rehabilitate and support persons with hearing loss through the health system.[10] In order to do so, it has focused on evidence-based advocacy with the aim of raising awareness on this issue among policy makers, professionals, and civil society. It has also worked to provide guidance to countries, through resource materials and technical inputs, for development, implementation, and monitoring of national strategies to make ear and hearing care accessible for all.

Advocacy efforts of WHO in this field have centered around the World Hearing Day, which is observed on March 3. Since 2013, WHO has proposed the theme and supported this with evidence-based messages and advocacy materials targeting policy-makers, professionals, and civil society. Many countries and partner organizations, as well as individuals have joined this advocacy effort by organizing a variety of activities, sharing materials and engaging with media.[11]

It is important that raised awareness is translated into policy and action at country and community levels. In order to catalyze this, WHO has organized numerous consultations in its different regions. Such consultations often engage with ministries of health and bring them together with professionals, academics, and civil society networks from different countries. This provides an opportunity for sensitizing all stakeholders on the principles of ear and hearing care, while facilitating the exchange of ideas and networking. In recent years, the program for prevention of deafness and hearing loss has also engaged with ministries of health in different countries to support them in strategy development and implementation for ear and hearing care.

Providing countries with standardized and evidence-based recommendations and guidance documents is a key aspect of WHO's work. These include training resources, planning templates, sharing of good practices, and more. WHO has developed many such resources that are commonly referred to and used by countries while planning and delivering ear and hearing care (**Fig. 3**).

The WHO program also needs to respond to emerging issues. In 2015, it identified unsafe listening practices among youth as a big threat to hearing health due to its widespread prevalence and the fact that most of those at risk are young individuals with potentially many years of healthy life ahead. In response to this, WHO launched the Make Listening Safe initiative in 2015 with the aim reducing the risk of hearing loss posed by unsafe exposure to sounds in recreational settings.[7]

GLOBAL HEALTH COMMUNITY ADOPTS A RESOLUTION ON HEARING LOSS

An outcome of advocacy efforts was that in May 2015, the World Health Assembly raised the issue of hearing loss and highlighted the need for a new resolution in order to accelerate work in this area. Following this call, a resolution on prevention of deafness and hearing loss was discussed and unanimously adopted by the World Health

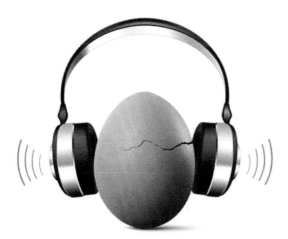

Make Listening Safe

Fig. 3. Logo for WHO's initiative to make listening safe. (*From* WHO Department for Management of NCDS, Disability, Violence and Injury Prevention (NVI). Make listening safe: prevention of blindness and deafness. World Health Organization (WHO). Available at: http://www.who.int/pbd/deafness/activities/MLS_main_infographic_A4_lowres_for_web.pdf?ua=1; with permission.)

Assembly in 2017 (WHA70.13).[12] This newly adopted resolution points to the importance of addressing hearing loss in order to achieve the sustainable development goals 3 and 4, which relate to well-being and education. This resolution urges countries to integrate strategies for ear and hearing care within the framework of their health care systems, as part of universal health coverage. It calls upon governments to

Collect population-based data on ear diseases and hearing loss
Establish training programs for human resource development
Ensure immunization coverage as a preventive measure
Establish screening programs for early identification and management of ear diseases and hearing loss
Improve access to cost-effective, high-quality assistive hearing technologies
Provide access to alternate means of communication for people with hearing loss

In essence, it provides countries with an outline strategy for addressing hearing loss. The resolution also calls upon WHO to undertake several actions that will support its implementation by member states and provide countries with guidance and technical resources required to act upon and implement the ambitious resolution.

FUTURE OUTLOOK

Based on the outline provided by the resolution, WHO plans to intensify its work in this field in the coming years. It has identified 4 strategic areas for work.

Evidence-Based Advocacy

In order to undertake effective evidence-based advocacy for prioritization of ear and hearing care, WHO plans to continue and promote observance of March 3 as the World Hearing Day every year.[11] WHO also plans to develop and launch a world report on hearing. The report will provide a global perspective regarding hearing loss and make recommendations regarding future actions to address this issue. As part of its advocacy and sensitization efforts, a learning module on ear and hearing care will be developed in collaboration with professional organizations. This module will be developed and implemented through training programs for professional skill development.

Data

In order to drive action for hearing loss, WHO plans to gather and collate data that can provide basis for advocacy and guide evidence-based policy formulation. Currently, it is developing a handbook on survey for prevalence of hearing loss and its causes. Epidemiologic studies will be conducted in identified countries across all regions using this manual. It also plans to undertake a global survey to assess hearing loss prevalence, access to rehabilitation and availability of human resources, and public health action.

EHC Strategy Development and Implementation at National Levels

This is key to the provision of ear and hearing care at the community level. WHO intends to continue providing technical support for the development of evidence-based strategies integrated within the health system framework. A toolkit of comprehensive technical support is under development that will assist countries in planning of EHC strategies, development of screening services, human resource training, awareness creation, and provision of devices and rehabilitation. Regional initiatives will be promoted and regional consultations organized to sensitize countries and professionals regarding EHC planning and provision.

Make Listening Safe Initiative

WHO will continue to drive forward this initiative in partnership with stakeholders. In the coming years, it plans to continue its collaboration with the International Telecommunications Union (ITU) to launch the global standards for safe listening devices, raise awareness through a public health campaign on safe listening, and recommend a regulatory framework for control of recreational sound exposure.

IMPORTANCE OF COORDINATED GLOBAL ACTION

WHO's actions can provide some visibility to the often-ignored subject of ear and hearing problems. However, WHO's efforts can only be a part of a greater plan. The collective responsibility of shaping the future of the hearing care agenda lies with all stakeholders in this field and has to be led by ear and hearing professionals, who need to move forward as a collective entity, sharing a single vision, with each one contributing to the whole.

In practical terms, it means that researchers need to ask themselves about the translation of their research findings to the larger population and its application in different resource settings. Teachers can imbibe and impart the concepts of public health as they apply to ear and hearing care. This will help ensure that future professionals in this field can have a holistic attitude toward service provision. Clinicians and service providers need to think of ways and means to make services accessible to all those who need it.

Most of all, professionals need to question themselves about the needs of and barriers to ear and hearing care and seek solutions to address these, with the ultimate aim that ear and hearing care can be accessible for all those who need it, across the world.

SUMMARY

Given the recent developments at international fora, there is a heightened consciousness about ear and hearing problems within the global health community. Stakeholders in the field of ear and hearing care, especially professionals, must capitalize on this momentum to raise awareness on hearing loss and ensure that it is integrated within health care systems of countries. There is an urgency for action, lest momentum is lost.

REFERENCES

1. World Health Organization: the global guardian of public health. In: About WHO. 2016. Available at: http://www.who.int/about/structure/global-guardian-of-public-health.pdf?ua=1. Accessed July 31, 2017.
2. World Health Assembly (WHA) resolution on prevention of hearing impairment [WHA resolution 48.9] In: WHO Prevention of blindness and deafness. 1995. Available at: http://www.who.int/pbd/deafness/en/english.pdf?ua=1. Accessed July 31, 2017.
3. Multi-country assessment of national capacity to provide hearing care. In: WHO documents & publications. 2013. Available at: http://www.who.int/pbd/publications/WHOReportHearingCare_Englishweb.pdf. Accessed July 31, 2017.
4. WHO global estimates on prevalence of hearing loss. In: WHO prevention of blindness and deafness. 2012. Available at: http://www.who.int/pbd/deafness/WHO_GE_HL.pdf?ua=1. Accessed July 31, 2017.

5. World Health Organization metrics: Disability-Adjusted Life Year (DALY). In: WHO health statistics and information systems. 2017. Available at: http://www.who.int/healthinfo/global_burden_disease/metrics_daly/en/. Accessed July 31, 2017.

6. Global costs of unaddressed hearing loss and cost-effectiveness of interventions: a WHO report. In: WHO prevention of blindness and deafness. 2017. Available at: http://www.who.int/pbd/deafness/world-hearing-day/2017/en/. Accessed July 31, 2017.

7. Make Listening Safe. In: WHO prevention of blindness and deafness. 2015. Available at: http://www.who.int/pbd/deafness/activities/MLS/en/. Accessed July 31, 2017.

8. Hearing loss in persons 65 years and older. In: WHO prevention of blindness and deafness. 2012. Available at: http://www.who.int/pbd/deafness/news/GE_65years.pdf?ua=1. Accessed July 31, 2017.

9. Childhood hearing loss: strategies for prevention and care. In: WHO prevention of blindness and deafness. 2016. Available at: http://apps.who.int/iris/bitstream/10665/204632/1/9789241510325_eng.pdf?ua=1. Accessed July 31, 2017.

10. Overview of WHO's programme for the prevention of deafness and hearing loss. In: WHO prevention of blindness and deafness. 2017. Available at: http://www.who.int/pbd/deafness/activities/hearing_care_programme/en/. Accessed July 31, 2017.

11. World hearing day: 3 March. In: WHO prevention of blindness and deafness. 2017. Available at: http://www.who.int/pbd/deafness/world-hearing-day/en/. Accessed July 31, 2017.

12. World Health Assembly (WHA) resolution on prevention of deafness and hearing loss [WHA resolution 70.13] In: WHO prevention of blindness and deafness. 2017. Available at: http://apps.who.int/gb/ebwha/pdf_files/WHA70/A70_R13-en.pdf. Accessed July 31, 2017.

Otolaryngology in Low-Resource Settings

Practical and Ethical Considerations

Susan R. Cordes, MD[a,b,*], Kevin Thomas Robbins, MD[c],
Gayle Woodson, MD[d]

KEYWORDS

- Medical missions • Ethics • Volunteer service
- Otolaryngology in low-resource settings

KEY POINTS

- Humanitarian medical missions require careful planning and preparation to assure successful outcomes and to avoid harm to the people for whom help is intended.
- Working in a setting with low resources often involves personal discomfort and medical risk.
- Scarce resources, religious beliefs, and local culture can lead to ethical dilemmas; therefore, decisions should be guided by the core principles of medical ethics.
- The best way for a novice to become involved in humanitarian outreach is to join an existing, well-organized program.

Humanitarian outreach appeals to physicians on many levels. It is an opportunity to see other parts of the world and to learn about other cultures. It can be an attractive escape from the pressures of a home health system, with the restrictions and coding requirements of third-party payers. Volunteer service allows for the practice of medicine without the burden of the business side of medicine; however, the core motivation should be a desire to make a difference, to share talents, and training to help others. Providing care in areas of high need can be incredibly rewarding—even addictive, but lack of preparation or unrealistic expectations can lead to disappointment or disillusionment. This can be particularly true for otolaryngologists, who are accustomed to

Disclosure Statement: The authors have nothing they wish to disclose.
[a] Department of Surgery, Indiana University School of Medicine, Indianapolis, IN, USA;
[b] Department of Otolaryngology–Head and Neck Surgery, Adventist Health-Ukiah Valley,
1165 South Dora Street, Suite C2, Ukiah, CA 95482, USA; [c] Southern Illinois University, PO
Box 19620, Springfield, IL 62794-9620, USA; [d] University of Central Florida, 6850 Lake Nona
Boulevard, Orlando, FL 32827, USA
* Corresponding author. Department of Otolaryngology–Head and Neck Surgery, Adventist
Healthy-Ukiah Valley, 1165 South Dora Street, Suite C2, Ukiah, CA 95482.
E-mail address: susancordes@att.net

working with sophisticated equipment and technology. During a humanitarian trip, personal discomfort, language barriers, inadequate equipment, cultural differences, and numerous unexpected obstacles can be expected. Even worse, there is potential to harm the people for whom help is intended. The fundamental principle of medicine, *primum non nocere* (first, do no harm), obliges understanding and preparing for the inherent challenges of caring for people in low-resource settings.

FORMATS OF HUMANITARIAN OUTREACH

- Full-time medical missionary
- Disaster response team
- Parachute team
- Visit to existing facility
- Teaching

Becoming a full-time medical missionary is a career decision—living and working in a less-developed country, most often under the aegis of a religious or other nonprofit organization. Disaster response teams, by definition, operate sporadically, so great flexibility of schedule is required from those volunteers. They must be able to leave their practices on short notice, perhaps for weeks at a time. Planned, short-term projects are more conducive to most otolaryngologists' practices. Parachute team refers to a group that goes to a remote location with minimal or no resources, bringing all necessary personnel, equipment, supplies, and medications. Such missions must be precisely planned and require substantial funding. In theory, working in an existing hospital or clinic with utilization of local personnel and resources should be less demanding, but working in a foreign facility also requires adequate preparation, including advanced coordination with local personnel and a detailed inventory of supplies and equipment. The American Academy of Otolaryngology–Head and Neck Surgery maintains a database of otolaryngology humanitarian programs, which may be used to identify an opportunity to join an existing program.[1] Teaching can be incorporated into all these models but also can be the sole objective of a visit. Education can range from teaching hygiene and first aid to community volunteers to helping local surgeons acquire advanced skills.

FACTORS DETERMINING LEVEL OF CARE THAT CAN BE PROVIDED

- Anesthesia
- Radiology
- Blood bank
- Pathology
- Critical care unit
- Specialized equipment
- Postoperative care
- Pharmacy support
- Audiology services

The level of care provided varies greatly, from basic outpatient screening and vaccinations to complex surgical procedures. Visiting volunteers differ in their skills and interests, but available facilities and local personnel largely dictate what can be accomplished. Some sites may not even have reliable electricity or running water, whereas others have fully equipped and staffed operating rooms. Embarking on a low-resource volunteer effort requires detailed knowledge of what is available at the site and what needs to be brought along, including personnel as well as equipment.

A successful low-resource volunteer effort begins long before reaching the host country. It is important to communicate in advance with host country providers regarding types and complexity of cases, number of cases, and local resources, and to thoroughly investigate important equipment, surgical instruments, supplies, and medications that are available on site. It should not be assumed that even simple items, such as silver nitrate sticks, vasoconstrictors, and sterile bandages, are available. A detailed list of equipment is important. It can take months to collect necessary supplies and equipment needed to augment a host hospital's limited resources. The process can seem at times like a scavenger hunt. Nurses in operating rooms and clinics are usually happy to save items that are being discarded but technically still usable, such as endotracheal tubes that have been taken out of a package but not used or sutures that are still sterile inside the inner packaging. Hospitals are often willing to lend surgical instruments or even equipment, such as electrocautery units, to physicians for such a volunteer effort. Most medical instrument and pharmaceutical companies routinely provide support to charitable work and most often have information on their Web sites about how to apply for equipment and drugs. The application and review process can take considerable time, so it is advisable to begin the process months before the trip. Americares (http://www.americares.org) may be able to supply some items, such as dressing supplies, sutures, and so forth. The American College of Surgeons Operation Giving Back program posts an online list of organizations that may be a source for equipment and supplies as well as programs that assist in delivering to low-resource countries: https://www.facs.org/ogb/resources/medical-equipment/donation-organizations (**Box 1**).

Any items left in the country as donations must be entrusted with someone who can ensure they will be used responsibly and competently. In particular, medication should only be left with a qualified health care professional or organization. Misuse of medications left by volunteer medical teams could result in illness or even death.

Anesthesia support is critical in any surgical volunteer effort. Unless there is confidence in anesthesia personnel at the site, a surgical team should include at least one anesthesiologist. Developing countries often depend heavily on anesthetists who may have less experience with difficult situations, in particular the airway. The types of cases that may be performed depend on the availability of providers of postoperative care after the volunteer effort is over. For example, repair of cleft lip and palate and some otologic procedures are well suited to parachute missions. Simple head and neck procedures, such as removal of branchial or thyroglossal cysts, are also amenable to short duration visits. More complex procedures, however, require local physicians to provide extended postoperative care. Removal of vascular lesions, such as angiofibroma or carotid body tumors, should not be attempted unless blood replacement is available.

Other available resources also influence clinical decision making. For example, the threshold for prophylactic dissection of a clinically negative neck is much lower in the absence of adequate follow-up to detect early recurrence or if radiotherapy is not available. The indications for total thyroidectomy are more stringent when patients may not have access to replacement thyroid medication. Absence of pathology complicates treatment planning, particularly for lesions that could be malignant. CT scanning, when available, is a tremendous advantage, but these expensive tests can be cost prohibitive for some patients.

PROFESSIONAL AND LOGISTICAL CONSIDERATIONS

- Political and cultural situation in host country (http://travel.state.gov)
- Malpractice coverage

- Need for medical license in host country
- Documentation of donated supplies and equipment
- Emergency contact in home and host countries
- Local customs, including attire in hospital and operating theater
- Communication among team members—mobile phones
- Voltage system—plug adapters, transformers
- Translation service
- Corruption

Political strife, epidemics, and natural disasters in remote places do not always register in the American news, and impending problems receive even less attention. Such information may be available online (http://travel.state.gov). It is important to be aware of the political situation in a host country and be prepared to adjust plans if there is an increase in security threat. For example, avoiding visits during elections or changes in government should be considered. Travelers may register with the US State Department to receive up-to-the-minute alerts and advisories (https://step.state.gov/step/).

In general, the risk of malpractice litigation in humanitarian outreach is low, but home country malpractice policies most likely will not cover in the event of an unfortunate situation. It is advisable to assess malpractice policies and consider whether or not to seek additional coverage. Licensing requirements also vary greatly from country to country.

Countries vary in how they monitor and control the importation of medical equipment and supplies. Often there is no oversight. Sometimes supplies and equipment are subject to taxation unless there is documentation of a charitable purpose, such as a letter from the host institution. It is important to assess the local situation and be prepared.

Voltage requirements and electrical adapters are easily found online. Research the voltage situation in the host country and the needs of equipment in advance to ensure critical equipment is usable. Communication with local personnel or with colleagues who have already worked in the region can inform a vast array of practical and logistical issues regarding local Internet and cell phone service. A cell phone may or may not function on the local network, and data and calls may be expensive. Furthermore, local personnel may encounter difficulty or expense in contacting a US number. Having mobile phones for communication can be essential to optimal functioning of the visiting surgical team. USB modems are an easy and inexpensive means of reliably connecting a laptop to the Internet.

Translation is usually provided by local physicians, nurses, or community volunteers. It is helpful to learn at least a few key phrases in the local language or dialect. Just being able to say "hello" or "open your mouth" or to express sympathy can go a long way toward building rapport and trust with patients. Helpful phrases as well as information on local customs and norms from more than 200 countries are found at the *Culture Crossing Guide*, a community-built online resource for cross-cultural etiquette and understanding (http://guide.culturecrossing.net/).

Although support staff are often not viewed as the focus of attention during activities, winning their affection and support allows for a smoother experience. Sometimes the biggest impact of a mission is the influence on the support staff by recognizing the important contributions that they make to patient care.

Corruption is a delicate issue. Some customs that appear to visitors as bribery may be accepted as courtesy or tipping. But truly dishonest practices can be encountered, sometimes are demoralizing, and sometimes present serious obstacles. For example, equipment and supplies have been confiscated by customs officials and then sold back to the same volunteers who brought them as donations. Unscrupulous local officials have been known to sell tickets to free clinics. Containers full of donations have been held up in transit until demands for illicit fees have been satisfied. It is important to keep in mind that the people being helped are not responsible for such actions and are in fact twice victimized by such systems.

Box 1
Pretrip checklist

Malpractice coverage

Medical license in host country

Immunizations

Prescriptions for common travel disorders

Antiretroviral medications

Review Centers for Disease Control and Prevention recommendations

Personal health insurance coverage, emergency evacuation coverage

Emergency contact person

Mobile phone coverage

Electrical voltage in host country

Political status of host country

Translator availability

Anesthesia services

Complexity and types of cases

Available equipment and facilities

Potential items to bring
   Flexible nasopharyngolaryngoscope
   Topical decongestant/anesthetic
   Anti-fog solution
   Headlight
   Otoscope
   Nasal speculums
   Bayonet forceps
   Laryngeal mirror
   Tongue depressors
   Alcohol pads
   Hand sanitizer
   Gloves
   Personal protective equipment/supplies

PERSONAL HEALTH

- Vaccinations: recommendations vary by country
- Prescriptions for common travel problems
  Coverage of bacterial gastroenteritis (ciprofloxacin or azithromycin)
  Coverage for giardiasis (metronidazole)
- Be aware of local or regional health concerns (malaria, zika, dengue, chikungunya, typhoid, yellow fever, and so forth).
- Make sure tetanus immunity is up to date.

- Consider medical and accident insurance that includes provisions for emergency evacuation to a developed country medical facility.
- Review Centers for Disease Control and Prevention travel recommendations for destination country (http://wwwnc.cdc.gov/travel/destinations/list).

Caring for patients in low-resource settings can be hazardous to health. The most common problem is traveler's diarrhea, which can occur despite seemingly scrupulous dietary precautions, that is, drinking only bottled or boiled water, avoiding raw vegetables, and refraining from street food. Most cases are bacterial, and ciprofloxacin is usually effective. Giardia is also common and responds to metronidazole. Norovirus, less common, is usually associated with more nausea, vomiting, and malaise, and recovery can be more prolonged. Whatever the etiology, fluid and electrolyte replacement should be ample. This may require intravenous therapy. Consider bringing along a few bags of saline or lactated Ringer solution. It is also important to remember that lakes and rivers may be infested with schistosomiasis or other parasites, and swimming in natural fresh bodies of water should generally be avoided.

Medical prophylaxis is recommended in areas where malaria is endemic. Malarone (atovaquone/proguanil) is an effective and convenient drug but also expensive. It should be started 2 days before the trip and continued for 7 days after returning home. Most other drugs require more prolonged administration before and/or after the trip. Even with medical prophylaxis, it is important to avoid mosquito bites because of emerging resistance. Insect repellant, mosquito nets, and long-sleeved shirts are recommended. The mosquitos that transmit malaria are active at night.

Immunizations must be up to date. The required/recommended shots for any particular region can usually be found through a simple Internet search, and the immunizations are often available at local public health clinics. The best way to assure being prepared is to make an appointment at a dedicated travel clinic. This provides a 1-stop opportunity to analyze and prepare for the risks of the region to be visited.

There is an increased risk of acquiring blood-borne infections in low-resource settings. The incidence of HIV is high in some populations, particularly in sub-Saharan Africa. Hepatitis C may be a high risk in other areas. Universal precautions should be followed just as at home. Consider bringing gloves from home, because the impermeability of locally available products can be unreliable. It is also important to have HIV medications available at all times in case an exposure occurs.

CHALLENGES

- Poverty
- Inadequate equipment and supplies
- Need exceeds capacity
- Lack of education
- Superstitions and reliance on traditional healers
- Record keeping

Even if surgery is provided free of charge, the cost of maintenance medications (eg, levothyroxine) or adjuvant therapy (eg, radiation therapy) can be a great burden. In some cases, a family may need to sell an animal or land to pay for care. In other cases, paying for care may consume funds needed for school fees or even food.

Equipment taken for granted in developed countries is often aging, absent, or nonfunctional in developing countries. Unless there is certainty regarding availability of a reliable electrocautery unit, bringing one should be considered along with an appropriate transformer if needed.

Supplies, such as endotracheal tubes and gloves, are frequently outdated, and disposable equipment is typically reused. This can feel uncomfortable, but it is a necessary reality in some settings. The quality of sutures and gloves may be substandard. Gloves may be thin and tear easily.

Degree of need typically exceeds available resources as well as the time allotted for the volunteer effort. Cooperation with host personnel is important to manage the expectations of patients who seek treatment and to triage appropriately. Volunteers should be prepared to manage the emotional burden of leaving untreated patients.

The education level of the population may be significantly lower in low-resource settings compared to that of more developed countries. Patients often lack the basic understanding of hygiene and diseases that volunteers take for granted, such as germs and nutrition. Patients and family do not always reveal their lack of understanding, so it is important to work with interpreters to ensure that information is transmitted effectively and comprehended.

Many patients have sought traditional healing and may have undergone treatments that are not only ineffective but also harmful. For example, in some parts of Africa, acute burns are coated with mud. Therefore, treatment may need to address the complications of traditional therapy as well as the underlying disease. Patients may also hold beliefs that affect their fears or even rejection of interventions. In some cultures, it is believed that biopsy of a tumor causes it to suddenly spread throughout the body.

Adequate record keeping can be a challenge in the developing world; however, collecting data during humanitarian efforts enables analysis of the success of the program to guide improvement of patient outcomes in future endeavors. Local records are sometimes challenging to read, with handwritten notes in a blend of English and other languages. Some sites have some form of digital record keeping, and advising and encouraging such programs can be another goal of the mission. The American College of Surgeons provides a Surgeon Specific Registry for this purpose,[2,3] or a data collection form (**Box 2**) may be used. Publication of experience can be beneficial to other humanitarian efforts.[4,5]

Box 2
Example patient data form

Name: _____

MRN: _____

DOB: _____

Gender: Male/Female

Procedure date: _____

Outpatient: Yes/No

Date of admission: _____

Date of discharge: _____

Location: _____

Role:
_____Primary surgeon
_____ Assistant
_____ Proctor
_____ Teaching assistant
_____ Co-surgeon

Assistant:
_____ Surgeon
_____ Surgical proctor
_____ Fellow
_____ Resident PGY_____
_____ Nonphysician
_____ Medical student
_____ Nonsurgeon physician
_____ No assistant

Pre-operative diagnoses: _____

Post-operative diagnoses: _____

Comorbidities: _____

Pathology: _____

ASA class: I/II/III/IV/V/VI

Emergency procedure? Yes/No

Procedures: _____

Wound class:
_____ Clean
_____ Clean contaminated
_____ Contaminated
_____ Dirty or infected

Complications: _____
Unplanned readmission within 30 days? Yes/No
Unplanned return to OR within 30 days? Yes/No
Death within 30 days? Yes/No

Abbreviations: ASA, American Society of Anesthesiologists; DOB, date of birth; MRM, medical record number; PGY, post graduate year.
Data from American College of Surgeons. Surgeon specific registry, Version 1.6.3.0. Available at: https://www.facs.org/quality-programs/ssr. Accessed August 31, 2017.

SUSTAINABILITY

- Partnerships with local practitioners
- Communication after the visit
- Return visits
- Education

The word, *sustainability*, has different meanings in different applications. In business parlance, a sustainable enterprise is one that continues to generate profits. In environmental discussions, sustainability refers to conservation of resources and preserving nature. In humanitarian outreach, sustainability means having a lasting effect on health outcomes, beyond the direct treatment of patients under care with that particular effort. The impact of outreach programs can be improved through collaboration and repeat visits. Providing education can effect lasting changes in the local health care system: teaching new knowledge and skills to practitioners, advising on ways to improve the health system, teaching care and maintenance of equipment, and so forth. The success of all these efforts requires sustained input, but the most sustainable endeavor is the education and mentoring of educators and leaders in the host country, so they can assume the mantle of improving health care.[6]

The success of long-term collaborative humanitarian efforts depends on the quality of relationships developed between hosts and visiting physicians. A good rapport allows frank discussions about gaps in care and knowledge and helps pave the way for future visits. Relationships are built on mutual respect. Host physicians respect the expertise and resources of visiting physicians. Likewise, visiting physicians must respect a host physician's knowledge of local systems and customs and be cognizant of the challenges faced and overcome by host physicians. Visiting surgeons should have a plan in place to care for and follow-up patients after a short-term mission trip. Good communication with host physicians ensures that patients get the appropriate and expected care and advice that may be required from a visiting surgeon. Return visits to the same site allow strengthening of relationships, long-term patient follow up, growth of the host otolaryngology department, and host physician career development. Collaborative research projects with host physicians serve the dual functions of improvement in patient care and academic advancement for host physicians. It is essential to comply with host country requirements for institutional review, and review may also be required in the home country of the visitors. Retrospective review is challenging due to lost or incomplete charts, so it is recommended that visiting physicians keep their own data while maintaining patient privacy. As discussed previously, the American College of Surgeons provides a Surgeon Specific Registry for this purpose. Information obtained may be publishable and may help to inform efforts at other sites.

It may be difficult to identify protected time for teaching in the midst of a heavy clinical schedule and may require sacrifice of time in clinic or surgery. Therefore, topics should be selected that are most valuable to host physicians, the target audience, and the patient population. Lectures are the traditional means of teaching, but language and cultural differences can reduce the impact. Interactive activities are more effective in adult education. For example, host surgeons can select and present a topic, followed by discussion. Case conferences, based on patients currently treated, can provoke lively discussion. Hands-on simulation is an excellent way of teaching technique. Cadavers are not widely available, but animal and synthetic materials can be used.

Much of the teaching occurs in the operating room. Early in the trip, evaluate the host surgeon's capabilities and tailor operating room teaching to the appropriate skill level and education/skill gaps. Inquire whether there are students and/or residents from the host country and their expected level of involvement. Expectations about visiting resident involvement should be established before the trip, because the presence of trainees from the visiting country may have an impact on the host physicians' experience. Visiting attending surgeons should be aware of residency review committee and resident training program requirements.

ETHICAL ISSUES

- Autonomy
- Justice
- Beneficence
- Nonmaleficence

Those who practice medicine in the developed countries do so in a highly regulated environment, one that includes an emphasis on best practice protocols and rules that protect patient rights. Also, the practice of medicine requires maneuvering within a structured system that encompasses administrative oversight, peer review committees, and detailed documentation. The same is generally not encountered in less-developed countries. The regulations and requirements that govern practice at home enforce the basic ethical principles of medical care. Humanitarian workers are obligated to follow the same principles in caring for patients abroad, but the administrative structure that helps health care providers conform to ethical principles is often lacking. For example, the Heath Insurance Portability and Accountability Act of 1996 regulations regarding sharing patient information only apply in the United States, but everywhere else in the world, patient privacy must similarly be respected. This includes never taking a photograph of a patient without permission and making certain to only divulge health information to people authorized by a patient. Patient photography may be an important means of documenting outcomes. It is also tempting for humanitarian team members to photo-document their experiences and interactions with patients. Patient consent for photography should be obtained and patient privacy respected, just as a visiting surgeon would in a home practice.[7] Photography consent can be incorporated into the surgical consent document, provided patients are appropriately counseled.

When situations arise that make it difficult to discern the best ethical actions, it is important to return to the basic principles. Autonomy dictates that each patient has the right to make an informed decision in consenting for treatment. Ensuring informed consent is difficult when patients lack the education to understand the science or when language differences restrict communication. The principle of justice is invoked in decisions of how to distribute scarce resources. This can sometimes conflict with the principle of beneficence. Although a treatment might have some benefit to one patient, it could be life saving to another. The principle of nonmaleficence is the basic tenet of all treatment, "First, do no harm."

Welling and colleagues[8] summarize the concerns that lead to unintentional harm during humanitarian outreach:

- Leaving a mess behind
- Failing to match technology to local needs and abilities
- Failing of nongovernmental organizations to cooperate and help each other and accept help from military organizations
- Failing to have a follow-up plan
- Allowing politics, training, or other distracting goals to trump service, while representing the mission as "service"
- Going where not wanted or needed and/or being poor guests
- Doing the right thing for the wrong reason

It is important to bear in mind that most health care providers in less-developed countries have learned to function in the setting of limited resources. They should be admired for what they have been able to accomplish. To help them advance the quality of care in their setting, it is necessary to work within the constraints of what is practically feasible. When participating in clinic activities, take time to observe how things are done. Each site has unique features of how patients are processed and evaluated and things often are done differently compared with home systems. Try to blend in without becoming an obstructionist and resist offering alternate techniques unless they truly enhance the process. Similar approaches are recommended when visiting the operating theater. Here, the process is usually even more structured, so simply observing how things are done during initial visits is best. Recommending changes and improvements should be reserved for later discussions and after developing a strong rapport with clinic and operating room staff. No humanitarian outreach is perfect, so programs should be evaluated for their value and quality of care. Maki and colleagues[9] published a tool for use in evaluating the effectiveness of humanitarian programs, and such assessments should be routine.

All physicians should demonstrate the highest standards of professionalism. The respect and compassion shown for patients, support staff, and families should be a model for practitioners who may be languishing in a frustrating system.

In a foreign health care facility, priority of needs may be different than anticipated. Too often, visitors bring equipment with the intention to add new innovations and treatments. When basic critical needs are lacking, adding new technology and procedures is like adding icing to a cake that has yet to be baked. A perceived priority of needs may be different than that of people with different cultural attitudes. Ideally, such issues are discussed in the planning of the mission, because adjusting for mismatch of expectations onsite can be difficult. Even worse, if local personnel do not reveal frustrations or disappointment to the visitors, this lack of communication can severely impair acceptance of and appreciation of the mission. Visiting teams should be well aware of what existing practices are in place. For some conditions, the local standard of care may be no care.[10]

It is essential to communicate with local administrative leaders, whether hospital directors, village elders, or local government officials. Make certain there is clear understanding of the mission and how it is perceived to be beneficial. Such encounters should be done with respect and sensitivity for these individuals. This type of personal interaction often opens doors and allows a visit to be more successful while establishing rapport with key individuals. Similarly, the initial encounters with the local peer physicians and staff are critical to establishing a rapport that supports a smooth working relationship. Avoiding showmanship, portrayals of superior knowledge and skills, and lack of understanding of priorities is important and leads to strengthening the relationship.

SUMMARY

Humanitarian medical outreach can be a rich and rewarding experience. It requires, however, careful planning and preparation. Not everyone adapts successfully in a low-resource setting. Challenges usually include uncomfortable living conditions, unfamiliar practice settings with inadequate resources, and significant risks to health and well-being. Joining an organized and well-oiled mission is the best way to become involved. Every issue cited in this article can be addressed through working within an established program, and the company of seasoned veterans on a trip can smooth the transition into an unfamiliar environment.

Perhaps the most difficult issue to face in humanitarian outreach is the limitation of what can be accomplished. The patients who could not be helped will always be remembered. The number who need care will nearly always exceed capacity. Diseases may be so advanced that treatment is futile. Some patients may refuse critical surgery or medication because of superstitions, lack of understanding, or lack of trust. A patient may show up with an emergency just as volunteers are leaving for the airport. The best way to mitigate such feelings of inadequacy is to work toward sustainable changes in the health care system, through fiscal support, return visits, ongoing collaboration and research, and mentoring the teachers and leaders of tomorrow.

REFERENCES

1. Humanitarian Efforts Map. American Academy of Otolaryngology — Head and Neck Surgery. Available at: http://www.entnet.org/map. Accessed August 31, 2017.

2. American College of Surgeons Surgeon Specific Registry, Version 1.6.3.0.

3. Sebelik ME, Zalamea N. Utility of American College of Surgeons Surgeon-Specific Registry for surgical outcomes data collection in low and middle income countries. J Am Coll Surg 2016;223(4):e129.

4. Jafari A, Campbell D, Campbell B, et al. Thyroid surgery in a resource-limited setting: feasibility and analysis of short- and long-term outcomes. OTO HNS 2017;156(3):464–71.

5. Sykes K. Short-term medical service trips: a systematic review of the evidence. Am J Public Health 2014;104(7):e38–48.

6. Fagan JJ, Aswani J, Otiti J, et al. Educational workshops with graduates of the University of Cape Town Karl Storz Head and Neck Surgery Fellowship Program: a model for collaboration in outreach to developing countries. Springerplus 2016; 5(1):1652 [eCollection 2016].

7. Holt GR. Ethical considerations of humanitarian medical missions II: use of photographic images. Arch Facial Plast Surg 2012;14(4):295–6.

8. Welling D, Ryan J, Burris D, et al. Seven sins of humanitarian medicine. World J Surg 2010;34:466–70.

9. Maki J, Qualls M, White B, et al. Health Impact assessment and short-term medical missions: a methods study to evaluate quality of care. BMC Health Serv Res 2008;8:121.

10. Hyder AA, Dawson L. Defining standard of care in the developing world: the intersection of international research ethics and health systems analysis. Dev World Bioeth 2005;5(2):142–52.

Using Technology in Global Otolaryngology

Robert Saadi, MD[a], Dana Goldenberg[b], David Goldenberg, MD[a],*

KEYWORDS

- Global access • Technology • Telemedicine • Robotics • Telesurgery

KEY POINTS

- Otolaryngology has adapted to, and even become dependent on, modern advancements in technology.
- Otolaryngology is particularly well suited to utilize telemedicine by virtue of reliance on endoscopic images and videos.
- Advances in robotics in otolaryngology have led to innovations in procedures of the oropharynx and larynx and may someday offer the delivery of advanced and specialized surgical care efficiently to remote areas.
- Correcting inequalities in global health distribution of otolaryngology services includes research and efforts in affordable distribution and use of specialty equipment.

TECHNOLOGY IN OTOLARYNGOLOGY

The field of otolaryngology–head and neck surgery has adapted to, and even become dependent on, modern advancements in technology. Application of technology in this field is widespread and evolving, reflecting the diversity of the subspecialties comprising otolaryngology–head and neck surgery and necessitating a wide range of skills and equipment. A driving force in the conception of the specialty as a unified field was the light-assisted technology used by early surgeons in otology and laryngology.[1,2] Visualization and surgical access are inherent challenges of head and neck surgery, and to overcome these obstacles, technology has steadily progressed from mirrors that reflect light from the sun to endoscopic, microscopic, and robotic surgery.

Disclosure Statement: The authors have nothing to disclose.
[a] Department of Surgery, Division of Otolaryngology–Head and Neck Surgery, The Pennsylvania State University College of Medicine, 500 University Drive, PO Box 850 H091, Hershey, PA 17033, USA; [b] Tulane University, 6823 Street, Charles Avenue, New Orleans, LA 70118, USA
* Corresponding author.
E-mail address: dgoldenberg@pennstatehealth.psu.edu

Otolaryngol Clin N Am 51 (2018) 555–561
https://doi.org/10.1016/j.otc.2018.01.004
0030-6665/18/© 2018 Elsevier Inc. All rights reserved.

GLOBAL ACCESS TO SPECIALTY CARE

Like the majority of specialty care, otolaryngology is most populated in the urban settings of the developed world. Lack of specialty services in rural settings and lower socioeconomic metropolitan regions can potentially pose difficulty in providing uniform health care. With respect to global access to otolaryngologic medicine, certain technological advancements and the use of telemedicine have become important, especially with regard to delivering care and follow-up to rural, remote, and resource-poor areas.

USE OF TELEMEDICINE IN OTOLARYNGOLOGY

Telemedicine refers to the use of technology to provide communication and patient care remotely through the transfer of information electronically. Certain fields are particularly well suited for this form of health care, including radiology, with the use of the Digital Imaging and Communications in Medicine, which satisfies the ability to interpret imaging from a distant location and communicate the results efficiently. Likewise, a complete otolaryngologic examination relies heavily on objective sources, such as radiologic imaging, audiometry, and otoscopic and endoscopic visualization, all of which can now be viewed, recorded, and transmitted electronically. Review of this data can be performed either via a live consultation, requiring a more concerted effort on behalf of the provider and consultant, or a delayed (store-and-forward) fashion, in which all relevant patient information, imaging, and testing are sent to a specialist and reviewed independently. The live interactive method, usually performed via video teleconference, aims to recreate the doctor-patient interaction of a face-to-face consultation, whereas the delayed method simply requires a response after review of information, suited well for diagnostic imaging, biopsy analysis, and other screening tests.[3] A study performed in 1999 by Sclafani and colleagues[4] demonstrated high rates of concordance with both strategies when reviewing flexible fiberoptic nasopharyngolaryngoscopy examinations, although it noted that the delayed method may rely more on higher-quality technology. Multiple studies have supported the potential of telemedicine to promote early detection by decreasing wait times for appointments, reducing unnecessary referrals and overall cost for patients, and increasing provider efficiency.[5,6] Along with increasing health care accessibility, telemedicine affords increased communication and distribution of specialized medical knowledge. As a surgical field, otolaryngology particularly benefits from the option to perform preoperative evaluation and postoperative follow-ups remotely, only requiring patients to travel for surgical intervention, which has been shown to be a financially beneficial and convenient method for safely monitoring patients in many situations.[7]

There are currently several areas in the developed world where access to specialty care is limited due to geographic and population concerns. Several such areas have already begun implementing telemedicine in the field of otolaryngology effectively. As with the inherent qualities of certain specialties like radiology to adapt to the telemedicine system, certain subspecialties in otolaryngology favor the format more than others, especially rehabilitation for vestibular dysfunction, speech therapy, cochlear implants, and management of middle ear pathology.[3] Otoscopic and audiological examinations for middle ear and tympanic membrane pathologies have been the most frequently used models adapted to this system. The Alaska Native Medical Center through the Alaska Federal Health Care Access Network project has reported success in implementing such a program for otologic patients with audiogram, tympanogram, and video otoscopy in store-and-forward telemedicine that now caters to more than

200 remote sites in rural Alaska.[8] Of 1458 patients studied, only 16% required referral to an otolaryngology clinic, with an estimated cost savings of $355,000.[9] Preoperative planning for tympanoplasty, mastoidectomy, stapes surgery, and myringoplasty was also found reliable between in-person consultations and delayed telemedicine.[10] A study performed by Hofstetter and colleagues[11] demonstrated that the average wait time for new patient referrals decreased from 4.2 months, prior to telemedicine access, to an average of 2.1 months over a 6-year period. Similar programs have been instituted for otolaryngologic services in Queensland, Australia, with studies showing cost-effectiveness as well as high concordance rates for preoperative diagnosis and management decisions in regard to tonsillectomy, adenoidectomy, and ventilation tube insertion compared with face-to-face consultation.[12,13]

Studies have also supported the use of telemedicine with speech and language pathology. Diagnosis typically involves perceptual features of voice and language as well as visual characteristics of laryngeal structures, both of which can be communicated electronically with ease. Investigators have found high concordance rates in diagnosis and showed comparably effective voice therapy could be delivered via teleconferencing.[14–17] Holtan[18] performed a study on videoconferencing an otolaryngology consultation during a real-time transmission of endoscopic examinations and demonstrated that the patient-doctor interaction is not negatively affected but rather that patient satisfaction benefits from increased options of participation with, and access to, a specialist.

Telemedicine has a special advantage in delivering health care to underdeveloped, resource-poor locations on a global scale. It presents the opportunity to provide advanced forms of technology integral to the field from areas where that technology is already in use to areas where the technology is lacking in the most cost-effective manner possible. Otolaryngologic pathology, especially hearing disability, is one of the most common nonfatal disabling conditions encountered in widely resource-poor regions, such as Africa, where health care high technology is lacking. A recent study surveying the otolaryngology, audiology, and speech therapy services in sub-Saharan Africa noted a marked difference in quality of health care provided in low-cost, low-income areas, specifically in regard to expertise availability and higher standard-of-care technology. Not only was there a marked shortage of specialty care but also specialists in these areas have become dependent on low-cost and outdated therapies. Of the 18 countries surveyed, a majority had either poor or no access to flexible laryngoscopes, operating microscopes, CO_2 laser, MRI and PET imaging, or radiation therapy. Ultrasound and CT scanning were more evenly distributed technologies but still lacking in some countries.[19] Thus, in conjunction with a paucity of otolaryngologists, the few available are compelled to practice lower-cost medicine and surgery than are those in the developed world. As technology continues to evolve in first world countries, this technological gap will continue to expand, potentially causing roadblocks for leading academic centers to even be able to provide guidance and support to the developing world. As such, it is important to recognize the influence of technology on standard of care in the specialty from a global standpoint. Efforts must be made in the specialty to conduct research and provide education in resource-poor areas to advance the field using affordable, yet evidence-based, methods.

TELECOMMUNICATION AND TRAINING

Much as telemedicine referral is an attractive concept in the field of otolaryngology due to patient difficulties in accessing specialty care, the technology in communication and data transfer proves important for disseminating knowledge from professionals to other providers in the field, improving training on a wide scale. Video teleconferencing is often used in communication between specialists, currently for use in grand rounds and multidisciplinary tumor boards. The extent to which this information can be delivered on a worldwide basis with the use of satellite telecommunication is paramount; this idea can be extended to even intraoperative consultation and resident training. One study demonstrated that outcomes for residents performing endoscopic sinus surgery while proctored by an attending physician in the operating room, compared with an attending from a remote site via teleconference, demonstrated no difference in clinical outcomes. The latter even improved educational outcomes for residents when there was an absence of attending physicians physically in the operating room.[20] As such, the educational prospect of telemedicine is an intriguing one because it may allow for more inexperienced surgeons not only to deliver the same level of specialty care as those at an academic center when being proctored but also to use that experience to efficiently develop skills and become self-sufficient, increasing distribution and uniformity of care in the field. This is also important when considering multidisciplinary care required for some patients and the potential for coordination with neurosurgery or ophthalmology with real-time surgical telemonitoring rather than in-person, intraoperative consultation.[21]

Ultrasound imaging is one of the more readily accessible and inexpensive technologies found even in underserved communities. Although less accurate than when performed by a radiologist, ultrasound imaging has been found a useful tool in otolaryngologists' repertoire.[22] After only basic training, otolaryngologists can use ultrasonography with 83% correlation to interpretations by a radiologist.[23] Again, this basic training relies mainly on dissemination of knowledge and has the potential to be performed in conjunction with remote experts and simulation models using modern technology in an efficient and cost-effective manner.

ROBOTICS AND TELESURGERY

Robotic surgery in the field of otolaryngology is currently most focused on procedures of the oropharynx and larynx and, like the majority of technology developed for this specialty, was centered on the need for better visualization and access to anatomic structures that would otherwise necessitate larger and potentially more morbid open surgeries. The transoral approach was first described in 1951 by the French surgeon, Huet. In the early 2000s, Steiner and colleagues[24] and Holsinger and colleagues[25] described the use of transoral laser microsurgery, the major shortcomings of which were manipulation and deliberate dissection around corners with poor visualization. The robotic surgical system, the da Vinci Surgical System developed by Intuitive Surgical (Sunnyvale, CA) provided better access while maintaining fine motor movements during a dissection of pharyngeal and laryngeal structures. This led to the development of the world's first TransOral Robotic Surgery (TORS) program by the Department of Otorhinolaryngology–Head and Neck Surgery at the University of Pennsylvania. In 2007, Weinstein and colleagues[26] developed the TORS radical tonsillectomy based on the transoral technique. The newfound method was shown to provide comparable cure rates and significantly better functional outcomes, as opposed to open approaches.[27,28] The research conducted by the University of Pennsylvania was used by the Federal Drug Administration to assess TORS, which was approved in December 2009 with the da Vinci System for use in both T1 and T2 malignant and benign lesions. Since that time, extensive research has been conducted further investigating applications of TORS, including skull base procedures and obstructive sleep apnea, continuing to transform and innovate the avenues with which patients may be better cared for.[29,30] In recent years, research has been conducted on the new Flex Robotic System (Medrobotics, Raynham, MA), an adaptation of the minimally invasive robotic surgery initially conceived by Carnegie Mellon University, for use in TORS. The system uses a snakelike robotic arm with endoscopy and flexible tools that have 102 degrees-of-freedom, capable of steering a nonlinear, self-supported path. It has since been shown effective even for visualization and access of supraglottic and total laryngectomies.[31]

With major advances in communications technology and robotic surgery, the concept of telemedicine can be further expounded on to its logical conclusion of telesurgery, or surgical procedures performed by experts in a remote location. This concept offers the delivery of advanced and specialized surgical care efficiently to remote areas and has been shown feasible even with current technology.[32] Costs are still prohibitive, requiring multimillion-dollar robots and links to high-speed data transfer technology in the underserved populations that are in need of aid.[29]

LOGISTICS OF TELEMEDICINE

The distribution of new technology throughout the world is dictated heavily by markets and regulations. In the United States, there is a strong push for new, state-of-the-art technology, including TORS and fiberoptic delivery systems for laser-assisted surgery. The technology is funded and integrated into standard of care, often prior to extensive evidence of long-term benefit. Even other developed countries, such as the United Kingdom and Australia, do not exhibit the same high levels of research and market-driven funding.[33] The history of robotic surgery in the field of otolaryngology has gone from preclinical trials to clinical implementation in less than 10 years.[29] As such, it is important to remain cognizant of evidence-based medicine in evaluating new technologies and procedures and to differentiate which technologies and procedures have appropriate data to be considered standard of care. New and expensive technologies that remain research and commercial endeavors under investigation may especially not be appropriate in resource-constrained regions where specialty care is limited. Furthermore, there will always be an inherent struggle between two noble but differing goals of delivering individualized, personal care to individual patients and delivering standardized, affordable, and uniform care to populations of patients regardless of location.[34–36]

SUMMARY

The history of technology in otolaryngology is as inspiring as it is exciting for the potential of the specialty to continue to provide new and improved care to patients. The specialty is defined by complex anatomy and often difficult surgical access, and professionals in this field have embraced this challenge by continually striving for the least invasive means possible for precise articulation of this occult anatomy. As is common with any groundbreaking innovation, some technological progress may be met with significant resistance prior to its adoption into standard practice.[34] The goal, however, should be to continue to strive toward innovation, superior patient outcomes, and widespread, uniform access to specialty care. Otolaryngology is a new specialty that is heavily centered in resource-rich academic centers, but the pathology treated is not limited to such areas. As such, it is a responsibility to pursue avenues for making affordable and effective care available on a global scale. Telemedicine is perhaps one of the best ways for extending the reach to remote and underserved locations and is particularly well suited for such a technology-adept specialty. Correcting the inequality in global health distribution of otolaryngology services lies also with the research into affordable distribution and use of specialty equipment and expertise as well as the development of new standards of practice to promote the interests of both the resource-rich and the underserved communities.

REFERENCES

1. Youngs R, Fisher E, Hussain M, et al. Technology and ENT. J Laryngol Otol 2016; 130:111.
2. Mozaffari M, Fishman JM, Tolley NS. How advances in light technology have shaped ENT. J Laryngol Otol 2016;130:112–5.
3. Holtel MR, Burgess LPA. Telemedicine in otolaryngology. Otolaryngol Clin North Am 2002;35:1263–81.
4. Sclafani AP, Heneghan C, Ginsburg J, et al. Teleconsultation in otolaryngology: live versus store and forward consultations. Otolaryngol Head Neck Surg 1999; 120:62–72.
5. Garritano FG, Goldenberg D. Successful telemedicine programs in otolaryngology. Otolaryngol Clin North Am 2011;44:1259–74.
6. Goldenberg D, Wenig BL. Telemedicine in otolaryngology. Am J Otolaryngol 2002;23:35–43.
7. Urquhart AC, Antoniotti NM, Berg RL. Telemedicine-An efficient and cost-effective approach in parathyroid surgery. Laryngoscope 2011;121:1422–5.
8. Kokesh J, Ferguson AS, Patricoski C, et al. Digital images for postsurgical follow-up of tympanostomy tubes in remote Alaska. Otolaryngol Head Neck Surg 2008;139:87–93.
9. Kokesh J, Ferguson AS, Patricoski C, et al. Traveling an Audiologist to provide otolaryngology care using store-and-forward telemedicine. Telemed J E Health 2009;15:758–63.
10. Kokesh J, Ferguson AS, Patricoski C. Preoperative planning for ear surgery using store-and-forward telemedicine. Otolaryngol Head Neck Surg 2010;143:253–7.
11. Hofstetter PJ, Kokesh J, Ferguson AS, et al. The impact of telehealth on wait time for ENT specialty care. Telemed J E Health 2010;16:551–6.
12. Smith AC, Scuffham P, Wootton R. The costs and potential savings of a novel tele-paediatric service in Queensland. BMC Health Serv Res 2007;7:35.
13. Smith AC, Dowthwaite S, Agnew J, et al. Concordance between real-time telemedicine assessments and face-to-face consultations in paediatric otolaryngology. Med J Aust 2008;188:457–60.
14. Mashima P, Birkmire-Peters D, Syms M, et al. Telehealth: voice therapy using telecommunications technology. Am J Speech Lang Pathol 2003;12:432–9.
15. Mashima PA, Brown JE. Remote management of voice and swallowing disorders. Otolaryngol Clin North Am 2011;44:1305–16.
16. Molini-Avejonas DR, Rondon-Melo S, Amato CA, et al. A systematic review of the use of telehealth in speech, language and hearing sciences. J Telemed Telecare 2015;21:367–76.
17. Duffy JR, Werven GW, Aronson AE. Telemedicine and the diagnosis of speech and language disorders. Mayo Clin Proc 1997;72:1116–22.
18. Holtan A. Patient reactions to specialist telemedicine consultations-a sociological approach. J Telemed Telecare 1998;4:206–13.
19. Fagan JJ, Jacobs M. Survey of ENT services in Africa: need for a comprehensive intervention. Glob Health Action 2009;2:1–7.
20. Burgess LPA, Holtel MR, Syms MJ, et al. Overview of telemedicine applications for otolaryngology. Laryngoscope 1999;109:1433–7.

21. Camara JG, Zabala RR, Henson RD, et al. Teleophthalmology: the use of real-time telementoring to remove an orbital tumor. Ophthalmology 2000;107:1468–71.
22. Bumpous JM, Randolph GW. The expanding utility of office-based ultrasound for the head and neck surgeon. Ultrasound Clin 2012;7:191–5.
23. Badran K, Jani P, Berman L. Otolaryngologist-performed head and neck ultrasound: outcomes and challenges in learning the technique. J Laryngol Otol 2014;128:447–53.
24. Steiner W, Fierek O, Ambrosch P, et al. Transoral laser microsurgery for squamous cell carcinoma of the base of the tongue. Arch Otolaryngol Head Neck Surg 2003;129:36–43.
25. Holsinger FC, McWhorter AJ, Ménard M, et al. Transoral lateral oropharyngectomy for squamous cell carcinoma of the tonsillar region: I. Technique, complications, and functional results. Arch Otolaryngol Head Neck Surg 2005;131:583–91.
26. Weinstein GS, O'Malley BW, Snyder W, et al. Transoral robotic surgery: radical tonsillectomy. Arch Otolaryngol Head Neck Surg 2007;133:1220–6.
27. Hockstein NG, O'Malley BW, Weinstein GS. Assessment of intraoperative safety in transoral robotic surgery. Laryngoscope 2006;116:165–8.
28. Moore EJ, Olsen KD, Kasperbauer JL. Transoral robotic surgery for oropharyngeal squamous cell carcinoma: a prospective study of feasibility and functional outcomes. Laryngoscope 2009;119:2156–64.
29. Maan ZN, Gibbins N, Al-Jabri T, et al. The use of robotics in otolaryngology-head and neck surgery: a systematic review. Am J Otolaryngol 2012;33:137–46.
30. Byrd JK, Duvvuri U. Current trends in robotic surgery for otolaryngology. Curr Otorhinolaryngol Rep 2013;18:1199–216.
31. Funk E, Goldenberg D, Goyal N. Demonstration of transoral robotic supraglottic laryngectomy and total laryngectomy in cadaveric specimens using the Medrobotics Flex System. Head Neck 2017;39:1218–25.
32. Bowersox JC, Cordts PR, LaPorta AJ. Use of an intuitive telemanipulator system for remote trauma surgery: an experimental study. J Am Coll Surg 1998;186:615–21.
33. Carney AS. Global perspectives: assessing the impact of new technology. J Laryngol Otol 2012;126:S1.
34. Meyers A. The ABCDEs of technology adoption. Otolaryngol Head Neck Surg 2015;152:587–8.
35. Kokesh J, Ferguson AS, Patricoski C. The Alaska experience using store-and-forward telemedicine for ENT care in Alaska. Otolaryngol Clin North Am 2011;44:1359–74.
36. Newman JG, Kuppersmith RB, O'Malley BW Jr. Robotics and telesurgery in otolaryngology. Otolaryngol Clin North Am 2011;44:1317–31.

Educational Resources for Global Health in Otolaryngology

Melyssa Hancock, MD*, Michael Hoa, MD, Sonya Malekzadeh, MD

KEYWORDS

- Education • Resources • Global health • Otolaryngology

KEY POINTS

- As global health initiatives continue to grow, so will the need for quality educational materials and programming.
- eLearning and open education resources are expanding the global communities' access to educational opportunities and experiences.
- The evolution of online resources and the development of telecommunications have allowed aid organizations to incorporate telemedicine into their efforts to expand the care they provide for underserved regions.

OBJECTIVES

The first aim of this article is to serve as an overview of the current state of global education, including suggestions for easily accessible programs and opportunities for local health care providers in limited resource areas. A secondary aim is to provide a summary of key resources for those interested in participating in an otolaryngology surgical mission.

INTRODUCTION

Rapid advances in information and computer technology have equipped today's educators with powerful and innovative methods of disseminating knowledge. World Wide Web–based and mobile learning platforms coupled with open access resources have become increasingly used methods of education delivery. In the global health domain, the diversity of these modalities and approaches transcend national boundaries and allows for a higher standard of care than was previously available.

Disclosure Statement: The authors have nothing to disclose.
Department of Otolaryngology–Head and Neck Surgery, Georgetown MedStar Hospital, 3800 Reservoir Road, Northwest, 1 Gorman, Washington, DC 20007, USA
* Corresponding author.
E-mail address: Melyssa.hancock@gmail.com

Otolaryngol Clin N Am 51 (2018) 563–574
https://doi.org/10.1016/j.otc.2018.01.005
0030-6665/18/© 2018 Elsevier Inc. All rights reserved.

In addition, this globalization of education allows for the transfer of medical knowledge from specialists to physicians who work in more rural or remote locales. This article highlights the innovative approaches that have fostered improved collaboration and coordination of global health efforts in otolaryngology.

EDUCATIONAL RESOURCES AND LOW-RESOURCE SETTINGS

According to the World Health Organization (WHO), the highest proportion of the global burden of disease falls on regions that also suffer from physician shortages. This is especially true of subspecialty surgery, which is all but absent in some developing nations.[1] Major contributors to higher disease incidences include environmental factors, nutritional deficiencies, limited public health measures, and behavioral risk factors. Examples of increased otolaryngology disease burden include chronic otitis media, oral and oropharyngeal cancer, and thyroid disease.[2] The WHO estimates that chronic otitis media is a major contributor to acquired hearing loss in developing countries, with 65 to 330 million people suffering worldwide. The developing world accounts for 90% of the world's 278 million people with bilateral conductive hearing loss, yet only 1 in 40 people who would benefit from hearing aids has one.[3] The developing world also harbors most patients with cancer. Two-thirds of the worldwide burden of oral and oropharyngeal cancer is in developing nations. Higher cancer rates and poorer outcomes are correlated with more disadvantaged populations. Iodine deficiency resulting in thyroid goiter is estimated to affect nearly 10% of the world's population, contributing to the high global burden of surgical thyroid disease.[2]

With an increasing otolaryngologic disease burden and an insufficient number of trained specialists worldwide, otolaryngologists have a critical role in the development of public health programs, allied health services, and educational programs for the medical and surgical management of head and neck diseases. In addition, residency training programs have created opportunities for residents to work internationally. In one recent survey, 25% of US otolaryngology residency programs were found to participate in global health volunteer projects.[4] For these reasons, it is important to inform and educate future surgeons how to incorporate outreach otolaryngology care into their careers and to provide an overview of free educational resources that can serve to augment global otolaryngology health through education in low-resource countries.

GLOBAL COLLABORATION AND PARTNERSHIPS

There are several ways the global community can provide otolaryngology services, especially as it relates to surgical education. One avenue is through participation in a short-term medical/surgical mission trip or global health initiative, generally organized by nongovernmental organizations, academic institutions, and faith-based or charitable groups.[5,6] A list of organizations involved in humanitarian endeavors (otolaryngology-related or affiliated national society Web sites) and a select list of the most relevant humanitarian opportunities are detailed in **Table 1**. More recently, numerous organizations and institutions have begun partnering with low-resource countries to form collaborative training programs and research partnerships. These partnerships can improve access and quality of care, decrease the disparities in access to surgical care, and strengthen health systems.[7] The sustainability of any humanitarian program or collaborative partnership depends on more than just the provision of surgical services. Education is an essential aspect to successful global health initiatives, whether improving the ability of the global workforce to meet the needs of underserved populations or supporting those participating in humanitarian medical care.

Table 1
Select list of humanitarian opportunities by region

Region	Organization	Details
Central America	APROQUEN http://aproquen.org/en/	The APROQUEN Burn Center provides comprehensive care free of charge to children afflicted with burns and those with cleft and lip palate in Nicaragua. It also provides technical training for sister organizations across Central America.
	Baptist Medical and Dental Mission International https://bmdmi.org	Health care professionals, along with pastors and nonmedical volunteers, join together to provide quality medical and dental care and education in Honduras, Nicaragua, and South Asia.
	Cornerstone Foundation http://www.crstone.org	This organization is a US-based Christian charitable organization dedicated to providing medical care based out of Hospital Loma de Luz, a 40,000 square foot, 50-bed mission hospital in Honduras.
	Center for the Rural Development of Milot http://crudem.org/	Sends health care volunteers, including medical students and physicians in training, to provide surgical services based out of Hôpital Sacré Coeur, a Catholic hospital and educational center located in Milot, Haiti.
	Hospital de la Familia https://www.hospitaldelafamilia.com	Hospital de la Familia is a nonprofit hospital that has provided vital medical aid and health care in Nuevo Progreso, Guatemala. There are four to six surgical teams that donate time each year. Each team is led by a team leader and is organized at least a year in advance.
	Mayflower Medical Outreach http://mmonicaragua.org	This organization focuses on providing otology and general otolaryngology services in Nicaragua, in conjunction with a broader effort that includes construction and physician training.
	Medical Mission Exchange http://www.mmex.org	Free, online database of short- and long-term medical missions serving the Dominican Republic, Guatemala, Haiti, Honduras, and Belize.
	Medical Missions for Children https://www.mmissions.org	This organization provides free surgical repair of cleft lip and palate deformities, burn injuries, microtia, and head/neck tumors. Dental specialists, nutritionists, and speech pathologists also participate in surgical missions to increase the range of services provided to the local population.
	Medical, Eye, and Dental International Care Organization http://www.medico.org	Provides health care to communities in Honduras and Nicaragua through short-term medical trips.

(continued on next page)

Table 1
(continued)

Region	Organization	Details
South America	Foundation for the Advancement of Cleft Education and Services https://facesfoundation.org/	Endorsed by the American Cleft Palate Association to provide care for indigent, medically isolated patients with cleft lip and palate deformities in northern Peru.
	Flying Doctors of America http://ffdoamerica.org/mission-trips.html	Flying Doctors of America has flown more than 200 missions and provided free medical and dental care to more than 185,000 children, women, and men. Among the areas served are Mexico, South America, Central America, Caribbean, India, Africa, South East Asia, China, and Mongolia.
	Global ENT Outreach http://www.geoutreach.org/	Trains medical students, residents, physicians, nurses, and health workers to deliver comprehensive ear care in settings with limited resources.
	Global Smile Foundation https://gsmile.org	Volunteers provide corrective surgical and dental procedures to patients born with cleft lip and palate deformities, coupled with educational and preventive programs.
	Healing the Children Northeast http://healingthechildren.org	This organization arranges teams of volunteer doctors, nurses, anesthesiologists, and other medical professionals to go to less developed countries where they provide medical treatments and surgeries for children in need. Treatment of cleft lip and palate deformities is one area of service provided by this organization.
Africa	AMPATH Indiana-Kenya Partnership http://www.ampathkenya.org	AMPATH is Moi University, Moi Teaching and Referral Hospital, and a consortium of North American academic health centers led by Indiana University working in partnership with the Government of Kenya to provide otolaryngology surgical services.
	Kenya Relief https://kenyarelief.org/	Every year, Kenya Relief sends 20 short-term mission teams to work in various areas of medical and surgical expertise.
	Mercy Ships https://www.mercyships.org/who-we-are/our-ships/the-africa-mercy/	Mercy Ships is a global humanitarian organization that uses hospital ships to deliver free, world-class health care services, capacity building, and sustainable development to those without access in the developing world.
	More Than Medicine http://www.more-than-medicine.org	Medical teams composed of otolaryngologists, anesthesiologists, and pathologists, as well as nurses and speech pathologists set up surgical camps in Kenya, Nigeria, and Uganda, where they provide continuing medical education to regional ENT surgeons while treating underserved communities with free health care.

Otolaryngology Training at Kilimanjaro Christian Medical Center http://www.kcmc.ac.tz	Kilimanjaro Christian Medical Centre is one among the four Zonal Consultant hospitals in Tanzania and serves as a referral hospital for more than 15 million people in Northern Tanzania. Clinical and surgical otolaryngology services are provided.
Fellowship of Associates of Medical Evangelism http://www.fameworld.org	Through partnerships with Christian missions and indigenous churches throughout the world, seeks to aid underreached and underserved populations using medical evangelism.
Operation Restore Hope http://www.operationrestorehope.org/about/	Operation Restore Hope is an Australian-based surgical charity for less fortunate children in the Philippines with birth defects and deformities, especially cleft lip and cleft palate.
Palestine Children's Relief Fund http://www.pcrf.net	This is a humanitarian relief organization in the Middle East that sends teams of doctors to provide pediatric surgical services in local hospitals, and also provides training and experience to local staff.
Philippine American Group of Educators and Surgeons http://pageshope.org	This group of medical missionaries focuses on helping the poor constituents of the Philippines, especially children who suffer from birth defects, such as cleft lip and palate.
Resource Exchange International-Vietnam http://www.reivietnam.org/programs/category/ent	Sends a team to Hanoi, Hue, and Ho Chi Minh City to provide expert ENT surgical services and educational and training opportunities for local health care providers.

EDUCATION AND SKILLS TRANSFER

Recent evidence shows that surgical conditions are responsible for nearly one-third of the world's burden of disease. Extended cost-effectiveness analysis shows that simply providing free surgery alone provides great health benefits to individual patients; however, the sustainability of the mission also depends on collaboration with the local health care community and cultural awareness, education, and skills-transfer. Providing educational and training opportunities to local community members and/or health care providers gives them the tools necessary to operate independently and to provide appropriate postoperative care and follow-up.

Education and skills-transfer may be accomplished through on-site and long-term education and training. On-site education may include observation, didactic lectures, bedside teaching, and operative experience. The evolution of online resources, including digital media archives and the development of telecommunications, has allowed aid organizations to incorporate telehealth into their efforts to expand the care they provide for underserved regions[2] Communication with local providers through email and telehealth arrangements via various mechanisms (ie, Skype, Facetime, WhatsApp) can assist with ongoing education even when specialist providers are not available in the host country. Provision of surgical videos and personalized lectures can reinforce the education and training of local providers. Unfortunately, some countries lack the infrastructure to support these advancements, so it is important to confirm the availability of resources and identify barriers to long-term health care sustainability.

For instance, an outreach organization focused on diseases of the ear may include the following components:

- Training assistance
  - Hearing loss
  - Use of hearing aids
  - Clinical management of chronic otitis media
- Establish regional temporal bone laboratories
- Live surgery demonstrations
- Surgical training
- Surgical anatomy and disease-specific otolaryngology lectures
- Sustained periodic in-person surgical education

In-person surgical visits serve dual purposes: to assess the progress of the individual local practitioners and further their education; and to boost the confidence of these local providers to treat these diseases in the absence of the visiting surgical team.

When considering which surgical skills and procedures should be emphasized in resource-limited hospitals, the available resources and the desires and needs of the host medical staff and patient population must be considered.[8] Efforts must be made initially to augment local capacity to care for simple cases, with subsequent trips focusing on more complex conditions, which require advanced surgical training. Understanding that this process can take many years is also important, because surgical missions often require sustained commitment from volunteers over many years to be effective.

eLearning

As global health initiatives and humanitarian mission efforts continue to grow, so will the need for quality educational materials and programming in developing countries. The traditional classroom style of education that emphasizes lectures and teacher-centered forms of instruction is difficult to establish and sustain in countries with limited faculty and institutional resources. Distance education has attracted much attention in recent years as potential ways to meet these resource shortages.[9] Nontraditional methods for education, such as eLearning models, have become popular as an increasing number of "just-in-time" products become more sophisticated, interactive, and engaging.

The Internet has expanded the way information is created and exchanged. Learners can engage in educational opportunities that allow them to use and build on knowledge in real time while teachers can share information and disseminate educational materials across continents. This globalization of education creates a collaborative atmosphere where students and teachers have access to and benefit from high-quality educational resources. eLearning, defined as learning mediated by technology, includes the World Wide Web, intranet, and multimedia-based computer applications.[10] It includes all forms of electronically mediated teaching, such as:

- Interactive online modules
- Video teleconference
- World Wide Web–based workshops/seminars
- Electronic medical libraries
- Online consultations
- Computer-assisted instruction
- Virtual education
- Learning management systems
- Simulation-based learning

Educational content is delivered and accessed in either a synchronous or asynchronous fashion. Synchronous delivery occurs in real-time and involves simultaneous interaction of participants with an instructor through chat or instant messaging, audio or videoconferencing, or live webcasting. Other advantages include the ability to record and playback sessions, log or track learning activities, and to personalize training. Through this type of virtual education, global connectivity and collaboration opportunities are numerous.

Asynchronous delivery allows flexible and self-paced training without live instructor interaction. The information is accessible at any time for instant learning and reference. Popular examples include the following:

- e-Courses are available in the form of either computer-based training, which can be run on the learner's system, or in the form of World Wide Web–based training, accessed through the Internet. It also allows interaction among participants through message boards, email, and discussion forums. Offline computer-based learning is facilitated through CD-ROMs and USB sticks.
- Self-study materials delivered via PowerPoint, blogs, wikis, or well-written articles and write-ups, such as PDFs, are the most common and popular methods of asynchronous delivery.
- Mobile learning (mLearning) involves retrieving information and resources over a cellular network.[11] This approach uses mobile technologies as tools and platforms so that learners can access instructional materials remotely for just-in-time learning.
- Simulation and gamification (game-based) deliver experiential learning through highly interactive and engaging methods that often include complex graphics and three-dimensional components.

Combined approaches that incorporate traditional learning with an eLearning component are now being increasingly preferred over any single type of training.

Blended instruction supplements the eLearning curriculum through a hybrid of electronic and face-to-face or hands-on methods. Studies have shown blended learning to be more accepted and effective. Students prefer interactive learning compared with reading a textbook alone, and active participation with increased learner engagement results in better student performance and improved educational outcomes.[9] Another key benefit of eLearning relates to teacher satisfaction. Educators are able to optimize communication and learning through a continuous loop of activities with testing, grading, feedback, and measurable outcomes. The blended platform also enables the inclusion of cofaculty, mentors and course managers.

The advantages of eLearning in low- and middle-income countries are numerous. It is the most efficient and cost-effective strategy for educating a large number of individuals over a wide geographic area.[9] eLearning increases access to educational content into resource-constrained settings and among populations that may not otherwise have access to such training via more traditional, classroom-based methods.[11] Furthermore, eLearning may be used as a means of extending the reach of experts in remote areas.[12] Distance learning does not preclude traditional learning processes; frequently it is used in conjunction with in-person classroom or professional training procedures and practices.

Despite the benefits, eLearning presents several challenges in resource-constrained countries. Inadequate infrastructure coupled with insufficient information technology support may limit the usefulness of this type of learning. There are often substandard computer facilities where learners may have little access to computers. Issues with low bandwidth, slow speed, and low quality of visual outputs are common and are exacerbated by frequent power outages. Navigating cultural disparities is another major challenge. Educational content must be tailored to meet the specific needs of the country and culture, while also adapting the materials to the appropriate language and idiomatic meaning.[9]

mLearning

mLearning is gaining attention as a solution for delivering education to remote and low-resource areas of the world. This is an increasingly used modality in which Internet access is through mobile phone carriers, and education is accomplished in locations where computer access is limited. As wireless networks get stronger and mobile devices become more accessible and affordable, mLearning may circumvent the challenges of access to World Wide Web–based learning and computers.[9]

OPEN EDUCATION

The digital age has enabled the concept of open education resources, which are defined as "digitized materials offered freely and openly for educators, students, and self-learners to use and reuse for teaching, learning, and research."[11] Open Education includes resources, tools, and practices that are free of cost and access barriers and that also carry legal permission for open use.

Many organizations offer no- and low-cost eLearning resources to those working in lobal health care. These resources include educational courses and materials (presentations, videos, reading lists, visual aids, articles, podcasts), resource centers, and resource networks (**Table 2**). For example, the American Academy of Otolaryngology-Head and Neck Surgery (AAO-HNS) AcademyU is an online educational and knowledge resource containing hundreds of learning options presented in a variety of formats to complement different learning styles. Developed by leading

Table 2
Free otolaryngology-related eLearning resources

	Name	Details
Anatomy	Anatomy of the Human Body http://www.bartleby.com/107/	The classic Henry Gray (1918) Gray's Anatomy of the Human Body; online edition published.
	Human Anatomy: Head and Neck http://www.dartmouth.edu/~anatomy/HAE/HeadNeck/hn_index.html	Dartmouth Medical School produces this site, which includes radiographs, images, and dissection videos.
Pathology	Atlas of Head & Neck Pathology http://ent.osu.edu/atlas-head-and-neck-pathology/	An Ohio State Medical Center on-line catalog of description and photo microscopic images of head and neck pathologies, listed in alphabetical order.
	Atlas of Oral Pathology (University of Iowa) https://www.dentistry.uiowa.edu/oprm-atlas	This atlas presents multiple gross and histopathologic examples of important lesions of the oral cavity.
Physical examination	Head and Neck Exam, A Practical Guide to Clinical Medicine https://meded.ucsd.edu/clinicalmed/introduction.htm	A comprehensive physical examination and clinical education site for medical students and other health care professionals offered through the University of California San Diego.
	Head, Eye, Ear, Nose and Throat Examination https://www.med-ed.virginia.edu/courses/pom1/pexams/HEENT/	The University of Virginia Health System created this set of instructional modules and videos demonstrating physical examination techniques.
Surgical atlas	Open Access Atlas of Otolaryngology, Head & Neck Operative Surgery http://www.entdev.uct.ac.za/guides/open-access-atlas-of-otolaryngology-head-neck-operative-surgery/	This is a free operative surgery text intended particularly for those surgeons in the developing world who are unable to afford textbooks. Supported by International Federation of Oto-Rhino-laryngological Societies.
Videos	Broadcast Med https://www.broadcastmed.com/otolaryngology/	The company was first in the world to broadcast live surgeries on the Internet using its ORLive solution, which provides an intimate look inside the operating room.
	American Head and Neck Society Surgical Videos https://www.ahns.info/resources/education/	These surgical videos demonstrate free and regional flaps for head and neck reconstruction.
	Cyber Text Book on Operative Surgery http://www.entmasterclass.com/headneck.htm	Provides an organized collection of educational resources on every ENT topic found in the public domain on the Internet, YouTube, Google, and various academic Web sites, including videos and online lectures.
	Live International Otolaryngology Network http://lion-web.org/	The LION Foundation is dedicated to improve the knowledge, skills, and discipline of otolaryngologists and provide worldwide education including developing countries. Their site is designed to promote distance learning using modern videoconferencing technologies.

(continued on next page)

Table 2
(continued)

	Name	Details
Journals	Cochrane Library http://www.cochranelibrary.com/help/access-options-for-cochrane-library.html	Cochrane and Wiley provide free access to the Cochrane Library in more than 100 low- and middle- income countries. Access is provided by IP recognition removing the requirement for individual login information.
	HINARI Programme for Access to Health Research http://www.who.int/hinari/en/	The WHO and major publishers set up the HINARI Program to make >7000 biomedical and health journals available to health institutions in the poorest 109 countries.
	Geneva Foundation for Medical Education and Research http://www.gfmer.ch/Medical_journals/Otorhinolaryngology.htm	Provides a list of all otolaryngology-related medical journals with a link to the articles within that journal that are free or open access.
	ENT Journal https://www.entjournal.com	Free membership for all registered users.
	OTO Open: The Official Open Access Journal of the American Academy of Otolaryngology—Head and Neck Surgery Foundation http://journals.sagepub.com/loi/opn	Peer-reviewed, gold open access journal that offers rapid online publication of clinically relevant information in otolaryngology–head and neck surgery.
Guidelines	American Academy of Otolaryngology-Head and Neck Surgery Clinical Practice Guidelines http://www.entnet.org/content/clinical-practice-guidelines	Multidisciplinary clinical practice guidelines are one way of increasing implementation of evidence into practice. They can serve as a guide to best practices, a framework for clinical decision-making, and a benchmark for evaluating performance.
	Iowa Head and Neck Protocols https://iowaheadneckprotocols.oto.uiowa.edu/	The Iowa Head and Neck Protocols offer a brief and directed approach to diseases of the head and neck and act as useful guidelines in disease treatment.
Case-based education	Lieberman's Learning Lab http://eradiology.bidmc.harvard.edu/LearningLab/central.html	This is a set of brief case seminars, prepared by Harvard third- and fourth-year medical students.
Radiology	Interactive CT Atlas http://uwmsk.org/sinusanatomy2/index.html	This atlas allows for interactive scrolling through normal sinuses in three planes, and includes labeled static images, which highlight pertinent sinus anatomy.

expert volunteers, the materials are designed to deliver relevant and current education. To make this online resource available to international colleagues, the AAO-HNS recently initiated the Member + program, called AcademyU Give Back, which bundles membership and access to all content at markedly discounted prices to low- and middle-income countries. The development of OTOSource is underway; this single-source online repository for all otolaryngology education content will exist in an outline form and serve as a road map of topics, learning objectives, references, and education activity links. Stemming from the collaborative efforts of the AAO-HNS Foundation and Otolaryngology Specialty Societies, OTOSource will be made available as an open access resource.

Additionally, medical journals are available online to providers in developing countries through the WHO HINARI program, including more than 40 otolaryngology journals. Some publishers directly support education of the global community (eg, SAGE Publishing provides free or deeply discounted online access to select countries). Live International Otolaryngology Network (LION) is an online video teleconferencing network dedicated to otolaryngology. The site includes a regularly updated e-Library with a comprehensive collection of surgery videos, conferences, panel discussions, and virtual exhibition and conference halls. LION seeks to enhance "the continuous exchange of ideas and sharing of clinical experience from among the world."[12]

TELEHEALTH

Telehealth refers to "the use of electronic information and telecommunications technologies to support and promote long-distance clinical health care, patient and professional health-related education, public health and health administration."[13] This service uses a broad range of technologies and strategies to enhance patient care and education delivery.

The Children's National Medical Center (CNMC) in Washington, DC serves as an example of a successful use of humanitarian telehealth.[14] CNMC has partnered with regional and international hospitals (in Qatar, Iraq, Morocco, Uganda, and Germany) to provide long-distance medical care to children, mostly in the area of pediatric cardiology. Using asynchronous digital echocardiograms and live video teleconferencing, cardiologists have expanded access to care for children with heart disease. The CNMC has also used the same technology to host distance education programs and live video teleconferencing presentations to include hospital grand rounds in Iraq and Morocco.

A creative use of telehealth to augment an educational program is a journal club conducted between consultants and colleagues in Phnom Penh, Cambodia. Articles and presentations are distributed via e-mail; subsequently the journal club is conducted in real time using Skype, a software application that allows users to make video-conferencing calls over the Internet.[3] Likewise, Medical Missions for Children is an organization that provides diagnostic consultations between partnering physicians and patients in remote locations in 100 countries via its telemedicine outreach program.[15]

SUMMARY

Education is an essential aspect of the advancement of global health. Although there is no completely comprehensive list or resource, this article presents a select inventory of available educational resources to serve as a starting point. The combination of electronic/distance-learning opportunities and consistent intermittent in-person surgical training efforts with the intention of skills-transfer are critical to improving otolaryngology health in low-resource settings.

REFERENCES

1. Chung KC. Volunteering in the developing world: the 2003-2004 Sterling Bunnell Traveling Fellowship to Honduras and Cambodia. J Hand Surg Am 2004;29(6): 987–93.
2. Groom KL, Ramsey MJ, Saunders JE. Telehealth and humanitarian assistance in otolaryngology. Otolaryngol Clin North Am 2011;44(6):1251–8, vii.
3. World Health Organization. Chronic suppurative otitis media: burden of illness and management options. 2004. Available at: http://www.who.int/pbd/publications/Chronicsuppurativeotitis_media.pdf?ua=1. Accessed September 25, 2017.
4. Volsky PG, Sinacori JT. Global health initiatives of US otolaryngology residency programs: 2011 global health initiatives survey results. Laryngoscope 2012; 122(11):2422–7.
5. Boon DA. Medical adventure in Nepal. J Otolaryngol 1980;9(6):526–33.
6. Pham AM, Tollefson TT. Cleft deformities in Zimbabwe, Africa: socioeconomic factors, epidemiology, and surgical reconstruction. Arch Facial Plast Surg 2007;9(6):385–91.
7. Riviello R, Ozgediz D, Hsia RY, et al. Role of collaborative academic partnerships in surgical training, education, and provision. World J Surg 2010;34(3):459–65.
8. Boston M, Horlbeck D. Humanitarian surgical missions: planning for success. Otolaryngol Head Neck Surg 2015;153(3):320–5.
9. U.S. Department of Education, Office of Planning, Evaluation, and Policy Development. Evaluation of evidence-based practices in online learning: a meta-analysis and review of online learning studies. 2010. Available at: www.ed/gov/about/offices/list/opepd/ppss/reports.html. Accessed February 16, 2018.
10. Ruiz JG, Mintzer MJ, Leipzig RM. The impact of E-learning in medical education. Acad Med 2006;81(3):207–12.
11. Centre for Educational Research and Innovation. Giving knowledge for free: the emergence of open educational resources. 2007. Available at: https://www.oecd.org/edu/ceri/38654317.pdf. Accessed September 25, 2017.
12. Live international otolaryngology network. Available at: http://lion-web.org. Accessed September 25, 2017.
13. Health Resources and Services Administration Federal Office of Rural Health Policy. Telehealth programs. 2015. Available at: https://www.hrsa.gov/rural-health/telehealth/index.html. Accessed September 25, 2017.
14. Lavin J, Shah R, Greenlick H, et al. The global tracheostomy collaborative: one institution's experience with a new quality improvement initiative. Int J Pediatr Otorhinolaryngol 2016;80:106–8.
15. Medical missions for children. Available at: https://www.mmissions.org. Accessed September 25, 2017.

Global Hearing Loss Prevention

Clifford Scott Brown, MD[a], Susan D. Emmett, MD, MPH[b],
Samantha Kleindienst Robler, AuD, PhD[c], Debara L. Tucci, MD, MS, MBA[d],*

KEYWORDS

• Hearing loss • Prevention • Vaccination • Cost effectiveness

KEY POINTS

• Hearing loss is the fourth leading contributor to years lived with a disability worldwide, affecting nearly 500 million individuals.
• The prevalence of hearing loss is greatest in low-income and middle-income nations.
• Social and economic costs of hearing loss are derived from assignment of monetary value to years lived with disability and are greater than $US750 billion per year globally.
• Etiologies of hearing loss are multifactorial, and include genetic, infectious, noise-induced, ototoxic drug-induced, traumatic, immune-mediated, and age-related causes.
• Further cost-effectiveness studies are required to optimize resources and develop priorities based on need, existing infrastructure, and financial circumstances in individual countries.

INTRODUCTION
Epidemiology

Hearing loss affects individuals across all cultures; it is the fourth leading contributor to years lived with a disability worldwide,[1] affecting 6% to 8% of the world's population.[2] Moreover, the burden of disease is growing. In 1985, initial estimates of global hearing loss were placed at 42 million individuals.[3] Since then, life expectancy has increased, and societal changes have made hearing loss owing to excessive exposure to loud noise and ototoxic drugs more common. Infectious and other causes of hearing

Disclosure Statement: The authors have nothing to disclose.
[a] Department of Surgery, Division of Head and Neck Surgery & Communication Sciences, Duke University Medical Center, 40 Duke Medicine Circle, M150 Green Zone, DUMC 2824, Durham, NC 27710, USA; [b] Department of Surgery, Division of Head and Neck Surgery & Communication Sciences, Duke University Medical Center, Duke Global Health Institute, Box 3805, Durham, NC 27710, USA; [c] Norton Sound Health Corporation, Norton Sound Health, PO Box 966, Nome, AK 99762, USA; [d] Department of Surgery, Division of Head and Neck Surgery & Communication Sciences, Duke University Medical Center, Box 3805, Durham, NC 27710, USA
* Corresponding author.
E-mail address: debara.tucci@duke.edu

loss continue to grow.[4] These factors, coupled with improved technology to detect hearing loss, require health care providers to keep pace with a growing problem. The most recent estimates indicate that one-half of a billion people now suffer from disabling hearing loss worldwide.[1]

Worldwide estimates help to frame the significance of the disease burden. Understanding regional differences may also identify specific causes and gaps in treatment availability that should be addressed. In an analysis of 42 studies from 29 countries, Stevens and colleagues[5] demonstrated that the prevalence of both child and adult hearing loss is greater in low-income and middle-income countries than in high-income nations. These findings support the World Health Organization (WHO) estimates from 2012, which found the prevalence of disabling hearing loss to be greatest in South Asia, Asia Pacific, and sub-Saharan Africa.[6]

Impacts of Hearing Loss

Studies that describe the profound impact of hearing loss illuminate the effects not only on quality of life, but also on the physical and mental well-being of individuals. In adults, those with hearing loss may be perceived as cognitively diminished, less able, and socially incompetent.[7] This perception is not limited to a single social or cultural group. In both developed and developing countries, the unemployment rate for those with hearing loss is higher than for their normal hearing counterparts.[8] In the United States, hearing loss is associated with low educational attainment and economic hardship, including both low income and underemployment or unemployment.[9] In developing countries, people with disabilities, including hearing loss, are at a higher risk for chronic illness and infections, as well as behavioral problems.[10]

Nearly three-quarters of a million infants are born annually with a significant hearing problem,[11] and the consequences may be devastating. In early childhood, hearing impairment may preclude the appropriate acquisition of speech and language[12] and contribute to poor academic performance.[13] Furthermore, these children will have more physician visits, days in the hospital, and days out from school.[14] Those with profound loss or deafness require greater financial support for programs teaching sign language or other means of deaf education.[15]

The effects of hearing loss carry over into the teenage years and young adulthood. Teenagers and young adults with even mild hearing loss are more likely to drop out of school early or experience unemployment.[16]

Owing to the vast worldwide prevalence of hearing loss, it is not surprising that the economic impact is substantial. These effects are seen at both the individual as well as the societal levels. As mentioned, children with hearing loss typically have lower literacy than their peers, affecting their neurocognitive development both educationally and socially. These setbacks early in life can lead to an increased likelihood of unemployment as well as poorer job performance.

Hearing loss is independently associated with incident all-cause dementia, with the likelihood of dementia increasing with the severity of hearing impairment.[17] Whether hearing loss is causative or associative with dementia has yet to be elucidated. Regardless, hearing impairment may be a marker for cognitive dysfunction in adults over the age of 65,[18] emphasizing the need for identification and treatment in these individuals.

On a larger scale, hearing impairment in a greater proportion of individuals may affect the proficiency of the workforce. To achieve long-term economic prosperity, a country relies on the cognitive skills of its population.[19] With an increasing proportion of jobs depending on both spoken communication and high literacy,[2] a greater prevalence of hearing loss will inevitably affect the population at a societal as well as personal level.

Worldwide Economic Impact of Hearing Loss

A recent report by the WHO[20] estimates that worldwide unaddressed hearing loss costs $750 billion annually. Included in this estimate are costs to health care systems at $67 to $107 billion; costs of lost productivity owing to unemployment and premature retirement at $105 billion; societal costs, including results of social isolation, communication difficulties, and stigmatization at $573 billion; and, finally, costs of additional educational support to children age 5 to 14 years with moderate or greater hearing loss at $3.9 billion. Importantly, it is estimated that two-thirds of the costs to the health and education sectors occur in countries that are not high income.

Why It Matters

Demonstration of the health related, quality-of-life, and economic impacts of hearing loss underscores the immense impact that hearing loss can have on both the individual as well as the global population. It is estimated that, regardless of the etiology, one-half of all hearing loss in developing countries is preventable.[8] Studies that examine the comparative costs of prevention and treatment of hearing loss reveal the cost-utility of prevention. Even in 1995, the World Health Assembly advised nations to incorporate preventative measures for hearing loss, as well as early detection programs.[21] They reinforced this statement in 2017, also calling for improved access to affordable, cost-effective, high-quality, assistive hearing technologies and products.[22]

The goal of this article is to discuss the causes of hearing loss worldwide. By exploring these etiologies, we will illuminate strategies for prevention. We will also describe current treatment measures that can reduce the impact of hearing loss on individuals already affected, identify gaps in access to care, and summarize proposals to address these gaps.

Defining Hearing Loss

Defining the criteria for what constitutes a 'disabling' hearing loss is critical to accurately assess the worldwide prevalence. Additionally, this process helps to identify specific regions that should be targeted for resource allocation that may help to prevent and treat hearing loss. The WHO defines disabling hearing loss (averaged over 0.5, 1, 2, and 4 kHz) as more than 40 dB in the better hearing ear in adults and 30 dB in the better hearing ear in children. Discrepancies between estimates of worldwide hearing loss reflect slightly different criteria for 'disabling' hearing loss. For example, the Global Burden of Disease estimates include a hearing loss of 35 dB or greater. Hearing loss can also be defined by grade, which provides an auditory description for the degree of hearing loss. Grades include mild, moderate, severe, and profound and range from 26 to 81+ dB, such that an individual with mild hearing loss might have difficulty understanding soft speech whereas an individual with severe loss will not hear most conversational speech.[23]

CAUSES OF HEARING LOSS
Congenital

Although less prevalent than acquired hearing loss, the consequences of congenital hearing loss can be devastating. The incidence of severe-to-profound hearing loss differs between developed and developing countries. In the former, it is estimated that 2 per 1000 live births are affected, compared with 6 per 1000 in the latter.[24] That equates to more than 700,000 babies born with permanent hearing loss annually in low- and middle-income countries. Worldwide, the prevalence of severe-to-profound hearing loss is estimated to be 39 million. These numbers make hearing loss the most common sensory deficit and congenital abnormality.

Genetic and environmental causes contribute equally to congenital hearing loss.[25] Although there are recognizable and consistent causes of congenital hearing loss, the exact etiology is often unknown.[22] In these cases, prevention remains challenging. Syndromic cases should be suspected when children have the classic concomitant features. Treacher-Collins syndrome, in addition to conductive hearing loss, is characterized by craniofacial abnormalities hallmarked by midface underdevelopment. Patients with Pendred syndrome may have a goiter in addition to sensorineural hearing loss. Patients with Usher syndrome will exhibit poor visual acuity, hearing loss, and in some cases, vestibular symptoms. Waardenburg syndrome, with its highest reported incidence in Kenya,[25] presents with heterochromic eyes and moderate-to-profound hearing loss. The features of Jervell and Lange-Nielson syndrome include cardiac arrhythmias and profound hearing loss. Not all manifestations of syndromic hearing loss are evident at the time of diagnosis of the hearing loss. Depending on the world region, one might expect higher rates of syndromic causes secondary to varying rates of consanguinity. Consanguinity remains common among 20% of the world population, particularly in the Middle East, West Asia, and North Africa.[26]

Several genes have been identified as common causes of congenital hearing loss. The most common cause of autosomal-recessive deafness throughout the world is abnormalities of connexin 26.[27] The incidence of deafness attributed to connexin mutations has been shown to vary depending on the subpopulation. The high frequency of connexin-26–related hearing impairment in certain populations may be the result of the tradition of marriage between hearing-impaired persons.[28] This notion is further supported by the theory of assortative mating, which describes mating preferences related to similarity in social backgrounds as well as similar phenotypes, which may include hearing impairment.[29]

Infectious

Several of the infectious causes of hearing loss fall into the congenital/prenatal category (eg, cytomegalovirus [CMV]). Infectious factors, however, play a role in hearing loss at all ages. From a systematic review of the causes and prevalence of hearing impairment in Africa, it is reported that the most common cause of hearing loss in the general population is middle ear disease (comprising 36% of those with hearing loss).[30] In addition to otitis media, measles, mumps, cerebral malaria, and meningitis are all important contributors.

Although measles (rubeola) is considered eradicated in the United States—despite clustered outbreaks—it remains prevalent worldwide. In 2010, more than 300,000 cases of measles were reported, with approximately 125,000 deaths attributed to its complications.[31] Although the acute symptoms, such as diarrhea, dehydration, and high fever often receive the most attention owing to the risk of death, subacute and long-term effects include pneumonia as well as deafness. Contraction of measles during pregnancy can also result in hearing loss for the infant.

Mumps, another vaccine-preventable illness, causes a typically benign, flulike illness. In addition to possible symptoms such as parotitis, sensorineural hearing loss can result 4 to 5 days after the initial symptom onset.[32] Hearing loss owing to mumps occurs in 3 different ways. The most common is sudden, unilateral complete loss. The next most common is partial unilateral loss. The rarest form is bilateral complete deafness, with fewer than 50 reported cases.[33] The frequency of hearing loss as a complication of mumps infection varies from 1 per 1000 to 1 per 30,000[34] cases. It is the most common cause of unilateral acquired sensorineural hearing loss in children,[35] although there are no accepted theories as to why mumps infections predominantly affect only 1 side. Before the development of a vaccine, mumps infection was quite common, occurring in more than 100 individuals per 100,000 based on routine surveillance. With appropriate introduction and distribution of the mumps vaccine, the incidence has been reduced by more than 97%.[36] In regions without widespread vaccination, it remains a more common etiology.

Rubella, like measles, can cause hearing loss both in those who contract the virus as well as the fetuses of mothers who are affected. Sensorineural hearing loss is the most common sequela of congenital rubella infection, resulting from direct cochlear damage and cell death in the organ of Corti.[37] In the congenital syndrome, hearing loss may be the only overt manifestation of the disease. In countries where no national vaccination program exists, up to 10% of women are susceptible. In India alone, it is estimated that between 42,000 and 267,000 newborns per year will be affected.[8]

Toxoplasmosis, CMV, and herpes simplex infections also fall under the category of "TORCH" infections (Toxoplasmosis, Other—eg, syphilis, Rubella, CMV, Herpes). Without treatment, the prevalence of toxoplasmosis-associated sensorineural hearing loss can be as high as 28%.[38] Although CMV rarely causes symptomatic disease in the host, congenitally acquired CMV can result in hearing loss. Not only is CMV the leading cause of congenital infections worldwide, but in countries where rubella has been reduced, it is the most common cause of congenital hearing loss not attributable to genetic defects.[39] CMV-mediated hearing loss has been well studied in the United States, and Europe, but its impact is less well-characterized in low-resource settings.[40,41] Given the growing evidence of geographic and socioeconomic disparities in CMV infection, CMV represents an important etiology of hearing loss that warrants further study in low-resource environments.[42,43]

Nutrition

Emerging data suggest that undernutrition may represent an underappreciated etiology of hearing loss in low-resource settings.[44] There is a small but growing body of literature from epidemiologic and animal studies demonstrating that certain micronutrient deficiencies and acute and chronic manifestations of protein energy malnutrition, such as wasting and stunting, are associated with hearing loss.[45–51] Multiple mechanisms have been postulated for these relationships, including infectious and congenital pathways. In an example of an infection-mediated pathway, receipt of vitamin A in a community randomized vitamin A supplementation trial in preschool-aged children in rural southern Nepal conferred a 42% reduction in risk of young adult hearing loss among the group who experienced otitis media infections in early childhood. There is evidence from animal studies to suggest that gestational vitamin A deficiency may also result in congenital hearing loss, independent of this infectious pathway.[44] Across multiple animal models, gestational vitamin A deficiency has resulted in dose-dependent aberrations in inner ear development in offspring.[44] If this observation persists in future studies in humans, it would have important implications for hearing loss prevention through prenatal supplementation in endemically vitamin A–deficient regions. Similar to vitamin A, there is also evidence suggestive of dual pathways in the relationship between protein energy malnutrition and hearing loss.[46] As these relationships are further characterized, they may play an important role in hearing loss prevention in chronically undernourished populations.

Noise Exposure

Frequent exposure to loud noise can also result in hearing loss. As the world has become more industrialized, exposure to excessively loud noise has also increased. The lack of noise prevention programs and awareness of the consequences of excessive noise exposure occurs in both developed and developing countries, but is more prevalent in the latter.[52] In most countries, regulations specify that workers should not be exposed to a noise level of more than 85 dB for more than 8 hours daily. In a study of mine workers in Zimbabwe, where no hearing conservation program was in place, noise-induced hearing loss was present in nearly 40% of workers.[53] Noise alone may not be the only reason for concern in industrial workers. Animal models have demonstrated that, as the carbon monoxide concentration increases in addition to noise exposure, there is an increase in the extent of auditory threshold impairment relative to noise exposure alone.[54] Heavy metals have similarly amplified the risk of hearing loss in the setting of occupational noise exposure.[55]

Noise exposure affects not only workers, but also individuals who are exposed to noise recreationally. For example, even listening to an MP3 player for 1 hour can result in temporary changes in hearing sensitivity measured by audiometry and otoacoustic emissions, indicating that there is potential harm in listening to these devices via headphones.[56] In a setting of recreational hunting, there is wide variation in individual susceptibility to impulse noise and use of hearing protection. Individuals may sustain irreversible damage to the inner ear from just one or a few shots.[57]

Drugs/Medications

A number of medications can result in significant hearing loss. A summary of medications that have the potential for hearing loss is shown in **Table 1**. Important medications to consider on a global level are antibiotics, antimalarials, and chemotherapeutics owing to their increased relative ototoxicity.[4] In many of these medications, the benefits clearly outweigh the risks of hearing loss. Examples of such scenarios include the use of chloroquine for malaria, gentamicin for neonatal sepsis, and multidrug regimens for drug-resistant tuberculosis. The danger arises from a lack of awareness and monitoring of hearing, which can lead to overuse or misuse. The low cost and unregulated over-the-counter availability of gentamycin make it a common cause of iatrogenic hearing loss and an important target for hearing loss prevention.[58] A study examining the prescribing practice patterns of 64 practitioners in Bangladesh revealed that all antimicrobial agents were

Table 1	
Common medications with hearing loss as a side effect	
Class	**Example**
Antibiotics	Gentamycin
Antivirals	Ganciclovir
Antifungals	Amphotericin
Antimalarials	Chloroquine
Antituberculous	Capreomycin
Antineoplastics	Cisplatin
Cardiovascular drugs	Furosemide
Anticonvulsants	Valproate
Immunosuppressants	Tacrolimus

prescribed in inappropriate doses and duration, based on patient complaints.[59] This finding is further supported by a cross-sectional study in Nicaraguan children that suggests the high prevalence of gentamicin toxicity is owing to unrestricted access to the drug, rather than by an underlying genetic susceptibility.[60] Antibiotics are not the only culprits, however. Although chloroquine is often used in developing countries as an antimalarial agent, it can also be used to treat connective tissue diseases. This treatment can result in sensorineural hearing loss, tinnitus, imbalance, and other cochleovestibular manifestations.[61] The incidence of ototoxicity varies with age, with some data showing that the youngest are most vulnerable.[62] There are a notable lack of data from developing countries on the prevalence of hearing loss attributable to ototoxic medications. Further research is urgently needed to elucidate the extent of the problem and develop evidence-based solutions to address this preventable etiology of hearing loss that disproportionately affects low-resource settings.

Age/Presbycusis

Another factor contributing to the increasing prevalence of worldwide hearing loss is age-related hearing loss from greater life expectancy in many parts of the world. Most countries are experiencing a period of rapid demographic change, which is not simply limited to the expansion of population numbers.[63] Owing to its lower level of socioeconomic development, Africa is assumed to be on a much slower trajectory toward replacement fertility, the level at which each generation replaces the previous one without substantial population growth. The international incidence of presbycusis varies widely, but there is some degree of hearing decrease with advancing age in all individuals. An analysis of the National Health and Nutritional Examination Surveys from 2000 to 2008 reveals that the overall prevalence of hearing loss in patients aged 60 to 69 years was 45%, and in those aged 70 to 79 years was 68%.[64] As the socioeconomic status of developing countries improves, it is expected that the prevalence of hearing loss associated with aging will also increase, approximating these figures seen in the United States and other developed countries.

Trauma

Injuries that disrupt the anatomic structures of hearing, such as temporal bone fractures involving the otic capsule, may affect hearing. Traumatic brain injury has recently been associated with a higher incidence of long-term hearing loss. In a study spanning a decade, it was revealed that traumatic brain injury led to a significantly increased risk of hearing loss.[65] With the high burden of traumatic brain injury owing to road accidents in low-resource settings, it is possible that trauma is an underrecognized etiology of the increased burden of hearing loss in low- and middle-income countries.[66]

Immune/Sudden

Multiple immune-mediated processes also affect the hearing pathway in children and adults. Meniere's disease, which primarily affects the lower frequency range, has a widely ranging worldwide prevalence of 3.5 to 500 people per 100,000,[67] increasing with age. Sudden sensorineural loss, which can result in significant unilateral hearing loss, presents in more than 66,000 new cases in the United States each year.[68] The prevalence of autoimmune conditions leading to hearing loss, such as Cogan's disease, lupus, ulcerative colitis, and rheumatoid arthritis, is unclear, but it is thought that they account for less than 1% of all cases of hearing impairment.[69]

PREVENTION

Uncovering the etiologies of hearing loss allows for prevention strategies to target specific causes whenever possible. The WHO estimates that 50% of hearing loss can be prevented, either through primary, secondary, or tertiary prevention.[70] Primary prevention aims to prevent hearing loss before it occurs. The goal of secondary prevention is to detect hearing loss early to reduce its effects, and tertiary prevention seeks to mitigate the impact of permanent hearing loss. Often, the prevention of a condition is critical, because high rehabilitative costs can pose a barrier to care in low- and middle-income countries.[71] In such cases, primary prevention could eliminate the need for costly treatment.

Primary Prevention Strategies

Strategies vary for primary prevention depending on etiology. In all cases, the adoption of primary prevention strategies depends on increasing policymakers' awareness of the prevalence of hearing loss and its social, economic, and health consequences.[2]

Genetic syndromes will present more commonly in areas where consanguineous marriage is practiced, but avoidance of this practice may be difficult in many cultural environments. Widespread vaccination may result in the greatest worldwide impact on the incidence of congenital and early onset hearing loss. As mentioned, the burden of vaccine-preventable infections remains high globally. In India, it is estimated that congenital rubella accounts for up to 40% of profound hearing impairment,[8] and rubella is one of the major preventable causes of hearing impairment across many world regions. With proper vaccination of girls before child-bearing age, cases could be reduced substantially or eliminated altogether. Despite this knowledge, as of 2002 only 58% of countries had routine rubella immunization programs.[72] The high incidence of bacterial meningitis in portions of sub-Saharan Africa represents another vaccine preventable cause of hearing loss.[73] Limitations owing to both the cost of the vaccines and infrastructure for care delivery contribute to the lack of comprehensive programs.

The examination of the specific costs of prevention versus treatment can influence policy decisions on the distribution of resources in constrained settings. It is estimated that the costs of screening a child for hearing impairment are 20 times that of vaccination.[74] The Global Immunization Vision and Strategy, which is endorsed by the World Health Assembly and United Nations Children's Fund, sought to reduce vaccine-preventable disease mortality and morbidity by two-thirds by 2015 from 2000.[75] For more than 70 million children in the world's 72 poorest countries, this would have resulted in protection against many potential causes of hearing loss including rubella and meningitis. However, the costs to do so from 2006 to 2015 were estimated to be $35 billion USD.[76]

In addition to promoting vaccination, limiting the widespread use of ototoxic medications can aid in primary prevention. The most common cause of hearing impairment from ototoxic drugs is the systemic or topical administration of aminoglycosides.[77] Both public education and professional education for prescribers are necessary to achieve primary prevention of ototoxic side effects. Ototoxic drugs should preferably be reserved for cases when there are no alternatives. Importantly, animal models and early human studies have indicated that therapeutic protection from aminoglycoside ototoxicity may be conferred from the use of aspirin.[78]

Primary prevention of noise-induced hearing loss should be emphasized in all occupational environments in which workers are at risk. Outside of occupational exposure, road noise and personal entertainment devices represent sources of risk for noise-induced hearing loss.[79] In the European Union alone, approximately 56 million people are exposed to road traffic noise at a level thought to be risky to health.[80] In both occupational and social settings, educational campaigns to promote noise avoidance and noise reduction should be implemented. The routine use of hearing protection and regular screening for noise-induced hearing loss in at-risk individuals should be universally mandated by employers. Although the prevalence of presbycusis increases with advancing age, limiting exacerbating factors such as exposure to ototoxic medications and loud noises may reduce severity.[2]

Secondary Prevention Strategies

Primary prevention, although effective, cannot eliminate hearing loss entirely. The goals of secondary prevention are to slow the progression of existing hearing loss, prevent complications, and limit disability. Prevention strategies are particularly critical for pediatric populations; in developing countries, the greatest burden of hearing loss is borne by children.[2] By the time some effects are evident, such as poor school performance, months to years of a potential interventional window have passed. One method for early detection is the implementation of routine universal newborn hearing screening programs. In the United States, 93% of newborns were given hearing screening tests during the neonatal period as of 2005.[81] Without such programs, the age of diagnosis can be delayed until signs and symptoms of hearing loss become evident. Other than the United States, only 17 other countries have a universal newborn hearing screening program.[82] Limitations of these programs include a shortage of individuals who are trained to perform the testing, the availability of calibrated equipment, and births occurring outside of a health care setting. In addition, the paucity of trained audiologists in developing countries limits the availability of trained personnel to oversee the programs and initiate treatment when indicated.

In the United States, more than one-half of states also require some form of hearing screening in school-aged children. School hearing screening provides an important method for detecting the hearing loss that develops after birth and is particularly important in regions where middle ear disease is common. In Australia, for example, where the Aboriginal population experience high prevalence of middle ear disease, telehealth has been used for community-based hearing screening,[83] and national school screening protocol incorporates tympanometry in addition to pure tone screening.[84]

The early identification and treatment of otitis media may help to slow the progression of hearing loss or prevent its development altogether, limiting associated disability. Early treatment of bacterial meningitis can prevent concomitant hearing loss. A recent Cochrane review supported use of corticosteroids to prevent hearing loss and other neurologic sequelae in high-income countries, but not in low-income countries.[85]

Baltussen and colleagues[86] examined the potential costs of screening children for hearing disorders in China. Their study concluded that the health care costs associated with screening programs and hearing aid delivery were less in the primary care setting. Screening methods will vary depending on the country, and variances in methods do not necessarily make one superior to another. The absence of these programs in other countries may be due to the lack of evidence-based local guidance, and financial or human resource-related barriers.[87] Recommendations from the WHO include implementing programs with clearly stated goals, engaging accountable individuals who are responsible for the program, performing regular monitoring with a clearly defined protocol, and implementing quality assurance procedures to show when results are not consistent with expectations. Countries in which cost-effective analysis has been performed have shown that universal screening should be prioritized.

Early identification is also important in the elderly population, where both the prevalence of hearing loss and the incidence of dementia are high. The relationship between peripheral hearing loss and cognitive function is complex,[18,88,89] and is particularly challenging in the clinical setting, where it can be difficult to determine if decreased cognitive function is the result of hearing loss or age-related cognitive decline. Furthermore, hearing loss has been shown to exacerbate cognitive impairment.[89] When these 2 conditions coexist, it is common for hearing loss to go undiagnosed. The use of periodic screening may help identify presbycusis for those over the age of 65, who are known to be at an increased risk. Education of patients and their families by primary health providers can provide tools for identifying the often-subtle signs of hearing loss. When present, these patients should be referred for treatment to help avoid the deleterious effects of hearing loss, such as social withdrawal. In individuals with noise-induced hearing loss, early detection is extremely important to prevent further decline. Routine screening in occupational environments where noise exposure is common will help to identify at-risk individuals and provide appropriate treatment where necessary.

Last, the development of information and communication technologies (eg, telehealth, mHealth, eHealth) offers potential solutions to address health care challenges, particularly for rural and underserved communities in developing countries that traditionally lack access to health care.[90,91] Telehealth solutions may improve access to secondary prevention for better disease management, such as identifying and treating hearing loss in both developed and developing countries. For example, the state of Alaska has used telemedicine to enhance access to care in remote communities for the past 15 years.[92–94] Validation studies have demonstrated that digital otoscopy images are equivalent to an in-person examination under binocular microscopy. This essential finding facilitated the development of expert triage telemedicine for ear-related consults and has greatly reduced the need for travel for postoperative follow-up in remote communities.[95–97] In addition to telemedicine, recent advancement in mHealth-based screening devices have the potential to further advance access to care in remote environments where audiologists and surgeons are scarce.[98]

Tertiary Prevention Strategies (Treatment)

When individuals who suffer from hearing loss are appropriately identified, there are a number of treatment strategies than can be implemented, depending on the cause and type of hearing loss. These strategies include, but are not limited to, hearing aids, assistive listening devices, aural rehabilitation, sign language instruction, and cochlear implantation. In the absence of such interventions, children may never develop speech and language or the ability to communicate effectively.[8] Allocation of funding in both developing and developed countries relies heavily on the cost effectiveness of the program or intervention to be supported. There has been an increasing emphasis on cost-analysis and cost-effectiveness studies in recent years to prioritize use of limited resources.

Although surgeries and hearing aids are useful, it is also important to consider adjuvant treatments such as aural rehabilitation. Aural rehabilitation consists of a combination of sensory management, instruction, perceptual training, and counseling. The premise of aural rehabilitation is that simply improving audibility of sounds may not correlate with improved hearing perception and outcomes.[99] By combining the use of hearing aids with short-term audiological rehabilitation, the cost per quality-adjusted life-year gained can be cut in half.[100]

Hearing aids can improve outcomes for individuals with hearing loss. Unfortunately, in developing countries, less than 2% of people in need of a hearing aid have one.[70] As discussed, simply augmenting sound with a hearing aid does not enhance communication, particularly in children, and the allocation of resources is necessary for education and orientation to appropriate hearing aid usage. The osseointegrated implant, or bone-anchored hearing device, may serve to benefit those for which the conventional hearing aid does not work, such as single-sided severe-to-profound hearing loss or a draining ear.[101] However, owing to the limited cost-effectiveness data to date, the bone-anchored hearing device is not considered interchangeable with conventional hearing aids for these potential candidates.

Cochlear implants support a high level of function, with sentence recognition scores of 80% or higher for most patients.[102] This finding is supported by a systemic review from 2013 that found unilateral cochlear implantation to provide not only improved hearing, but also significantly improved quality of life.[103] Restricted access to cochlear implants is not limited to developing countries. In Canada, as the number of annual cochlear implants increases, access is expected to bottleneck owing to both provincial funding and access to surgical expertise.[104] Similar issues likely affect access in many countries.

The costs associated with cochlear implantation are not limited to the device itself. Implantation requires a surgical procedure, with associated operative costs, as well as close follow-up for programming and hearing rehabilitation. Cost-effectiveness studies have been performed in both developed and developing countries and, when consideration extends to discounted lifetime costs of the intervention, implants are cost effective in both high- and low-resource settings. Cost analyses in low-income countries are aided by the fact that surgical and medical personnel costs are lower in these countries, and children who are implanted earlier require fewer resources for education. In Nicaragua, the poorest country in the Western hemisphere, cochlear implantation is cost effective and compares favorably with deaf education in lifetime costs.[105] In Hong Kong, cochlear implants have been shown to have cost effectiveness greater than knee replacements, implantable defibrillators, and dialysis.[106] In a study analyzing the cost effectiveness of cochlear implantation in sub-Saharan African countries,[107] cochlear implantation was most cost effective in South Africa, the only country with a robust national cochlear implantation program, and the country with the highest gross domestic product in this region. Although not yet cost effective in some emerging sub-Saharan African economies included in the study, a sensitivity analysis that varied the cost of the cochlear implant showed that lower device costs could render this intervention cost effective in countries with a lower gross domestic product. The authors aptly emphasize that quantifying the cost effectiveness of health intervention can only be done within the context of the local environment.

Prioritization of Prevention Strategies

The development of primary, secondary, and tertiary programs for hearing loss prevention and amelioration may seem like a daunting task in very low-resource environments. However, even in impoverished settings progress can be made, and efforts built on as resources increase. A comprehensive strategy for addressing this burden should be developed on a country-by-country basis, with subsequent efforts building on what has already been accomplished. A new WHO resolution calls on governments of all member nations to integrate strategies for ear and hearing care within the framework of their primary health care systems.[22] Strategies for decreasing the burden of hearing loss according to per-capita income have been described,[2,8] and are summarized in **Box 1**.

Box1
Suggested strategies for reducing the burden of hearing loss according to country per capita income

Low-Income Countries

- Assess the burden of disease to determine major causes
- Develop an educational campaign for the general public, including healthy practices during pregnancy, speech and language milestones, the importance of vaccinations, and avoidance of consanguinity
- Develop an educational program for health practitioners, including office or field assessments of hearing, speech and language development milestones, ear examination, treatment of ear infections and cerumen impactions, the importance of vaccinations, and the avoidance of ototoxic medications and high levels of noise

Middle-Income Countries

- Institute universal newborn hearing screening
- Institute vaccination programs
- Work with the government and foundations to provide access to technologies such as hearing aids and cochlear implants
- Increase training of needed professionals, including otolaryngologists, audiologists, speech language pathologists, teachers of the hearing impaired, and trained health workers, and make services available in rural as well as urban areas
- Provide educational opportunities for all children, by whatever means they can be successfully taught

High-Income Countries

- Provide periodic screening of school-age children
- Ensure hearing aid and cochlear implant technology is available to all regardless of income or geography
- Ensure appropriate hearing health care available to all regardless of income
- Ensure proper educational resources available to all children
- Devote special attention to the elderly, who are particularly affected in developed countries; ensure that hearing health care is available regardless of income or geography; significant hearing loss in this age group can lead to depression and withdrawal from society and is associated with dementia and other negative health outcomes[108]

From Tucci D, Merson MH, Wilson BS. A summary of the literature on global hearing impairment: current status and priorities for action. Otol Neurotol 2010;31(1):39; with permission.

SUMMARY

Hearing loss represents the most common sensory impairment worldwide and is estimated to affect greater than one-half of a billion individuals. The estimates of people affected by hearing loss continue to increase, as do the associated costs. In the United States, costs associated with hearing loss approach $US175 billion each year,[109] despite the appropriate preventative and rehabilitative services available. Worldwide, these total costs are staggering when accounting for the economic and societal costs in addition to the burden on health care.

Programs to help detect hearing loss early and provide appropriate treatment are essential to reducing the disabilities associated with hearing loss. With nearly one-half of all hearing loss attributed to preventable causes, primary prevention strategies must be emphasized. Vaccine-preventable infections remain a key area for improvement. Multiple studies have demonstrated the cost effectiveness of preventive and rehabilitative programs, and a cohesive front is necessary to implement them on a global level.

REFERENCES

1. GBD 2015 Disease and Injury Incidence and Prevalence Collaborators. Global, regional, and national incidence, prevalence, and years lived with disability for 310 diseases and injuries, 1990–2015: a systematic analysis for the Global Burden of Disease Study. The Lancet 2015;388(10053):1545–602.
2. Wilson BS, Tucci DL, Merson MH, et al. Global hearing health care: new findings and perspectives. Lancet 2017;390(10111):2503–15.
3. Smith A. Preventing deafness: an achievable challenge. The WHO perspective. International Congress Series 2003;1240:183–91.
4. Arslan E, Orzan E, Santarelli R. Global problem of drug-induced hearing loss. Ann N Y Acad Sci 1999;884(1):1–14.
5. Stevens G, Flaxman S, Brunskill E, et al. Global and regional hearing impairment prevalence: an analysis of 42 studies in 29 countries. Eur J Public Health 2013; 23(1):146–52.
6. WHO global estimates on prevalence of hearing loss. 2012. 2017. Available at: http://www.who.int/pbd/deafness/estimates/en/. Accessed October 19, 2017.
7. Southall K, Gagne JP, Jennings MB. Stigma: a negative and a positive influence on help-seeking for adults with acquired hearing loss. Int J Audiol 2010;49(11): 804–14.
8. Tucci D, Merson MH, Wilson BS. A summary of the literature on global hearing impairment: current status and priorities for action. Otol Neurotol 2010;31(1): 31–41.
9. Emmett SD, Francis HW. The socioeconomic impact of hearing loss in US adults. Otol Neurotol 2015;36(3):545–50.
10. Groce NE. People with disabilities. In: Levy BS, Sidel VW, editors. Social injustice and public health. New York: Oxford University Press; 2013. p. 140–57.
11. Smith RJ, Bale JF Jr, White KR. Sensorineural hearing loss in children. Lancet 2005;365(9462):879–90.
12. Kennedy CR, McCann DC, Campbell MJ, et al. Language ability after early detection of permanent childhood hearing impairment. N Engl J Med 2006; 354(20):2131–41.
13. Emmett SD, Francis HW. Bilateral hearing loss is associated with decreased nonverbal intelligence in US children aged 6 to 16 years. Laryngoscope 2014; 124(9):2176–81.
14. Olusanya BO, Ruben RJ, Parving A. Reducing the burden of communication disorders in the developing world: an opportunity for the millennium development project. JAMA 2006;296(4):441–4.
15. Low WK, Pang KY, Ho LY, et al. Universal newborn hearing screening in Singapore: the need, implementation and challenges. Ann Acad Med Singapore 2005;34(4):301–6.
16. Järvelin MR, Mäki–torkko E, Sorri MJ, et al. Effect of hearing impairment on educational outcomes and employment up to the age of 25 years in Northern Finland. Br J Audiol 1997;31(3):165–75.
17. Lin FR, Metter EJ, O'Brien RJ, et al. Hearing loss and incident dementia. Arch Neurol 2011;68(2):214–20.

18. Gurgel RK, Ward PD, Schwartz S, et al. Relationship of hearing loss and dementia: a prospective, population-based study. Otol Neurotol 2014;35(5):775–81.
19. Hanushek EA, Woesmann L. The knowledge capital of nations: education and the economics of growth. Cambridge (MA): MIT Press; 2015.
20. Global costs of unaddressed hearing loss and cost-effectiveness of interventions: a WHO report, 2017. Geneva (Switzerland): World Health Organization; 2017.
21. WHA48.9 prevention of hearing impairment. Twelfth plenary meeting, 12 May 1995 – Committee A, second report. Geneva (Switzerland): World Health Organization; 1995.
22. Seventieth World Health Assembly update, 30 May 2017. 2017. Available at: http://www.who.int/mediacentre/news/releases/2017/vector-control-ncds-cancer/en. Accessed August 23, 2017.
23. World Health Organization (WHO). Grades of hearing impairment. Available at: http://www.who.int/pbd/deafness/hearing_impairment_grades/en/. Accessed August 23, 2017.
24. Olusanya BO. Neonatal hearing screening and intervention in resource-limited settings: an overview. Arch Dis Child 2012;97(7):654–9.
25. Nayak CS, Isaacson G. Worldwide distribution of Waardenburg syndrome. Ann Otol Rhinol Laryngol 2003;112(9 Pt 1):817–20.
26. Hamamy H. Consanguineous marriages: preconception consultation in primary health care settings. J Community Genet 2012;3(3):185–92.
27. Kemperman MH, Hoefsloot LH, Cremers CWRJ. Hearing loss and connexin 26. J R Soc Med 2002;95(4):171–7.
28. Nance WE, Liu XZ, Pandya A. Relation between choice of partner and high frequency of cannexin-26 deafness. Lancet 2000;356(9228):500–1.
29. Zietsch BP, Verweij KJH, Heath AC, et al. Variation in human mate choice: simultaneously investigating heritability, parental influence, sexual imprinting, and assortative mating. Am Nat 2011;177(5):605–16.
30. Mulwafu W, Kuper H, Ensink RJH. Prevalence and causes of hearing impairment in Africa. Trop Med Int Health 2016;21(2):158–65.
31. Simons E, Ferrari M, Fricks J, et al. Assessment of the 2010 global measles mortality reduction goal: results from a model of surveillance data. Lancet 2012; 379(9832):2173–8.
32. Hall R, Richards H. Hearing loss due to mumps. Arch Dis Child 1987;62(2): 189–91.
33. Bitnun S, Rakover Y, Rosen G. Acute bilateral total deafness complicating mumps. J Laryngol Otol 2007;100(8):943–5.
34. Cohen BE, Durstenfeld A, Roehm PC. Viral causes of hearing loss: a review for hearing health professionals. Trends Hear 2014;18. 2331216514541361.
35. Paparella MM, Schachem PA. Sensorineural hearing loss in children - nongenetic. Otolaryngology, vol. 2. Philadelphia: Saunders; 1991. p. 1571–2.
36. Galazka AM, Robertson SE, Kraigher A. Mumps and mumps vaccine: a global review. Bull World Health Organ 1999;77(1):3–14.
37. Lee JY, Scott Bowden D. Rubella virus replication and links to teratogenicity. Clin Microbiol Rev 2000;13(4):571–87.
38. Brown ED, Chau JK, Atashband S, et al. A systematic review of neonatal toxoplasmosis exposure and sensorineural hearing loss. Int J Pediatr Otorhinolaryngol 2009;73(5):707–11.
39. Manicklal S, Emery VC, Lazzarotto T, et al. The "silent" global burden of congenital cytomegalovirus. Clin Microbiol Rev 2013;26(1):86–102.

40. Goderis J, Keymeulen A, Smets K, et al. Hearing in children with congenital cytomegalovirus infection: results of a longitudinal study. J Pediatr 2016;172:110–5.e2.

41. Grosse SD, Ross DS, Dollard SC. Congenital cytomegalovirus (CMV) infection as a cause of permanent bilateral hearing loss: a quantitative assessment. J Clin Virol 2008;41(2):57–62.

42. Lantos P, Hoffman K, Permar S, et al. Geographic disparities in cytomegalovirus infection during pregnancy. J Pediatric Infect Dis Soc 2017;6(3):e55–61.

43. Lantos PM, Permar SR, Hoffman K, et al. The excess burden of cytomegalovirus in African American communities: a geospatial analysis. Open Forum Infect Dis 2015;2(4):ofv180.

44. Emmett SD, West KP. Gestational vitamin A deficiency: a novel cause of sensorineural hearing loss in the developing world? Med Hypotheses 2014;82(1):6–10.

45. Schmitz J, West KP, Khatry SK, et al. Vitamin A supplementation in preschool children and risk of hearing loss as adolescents and young adults in rural Nepal: randomised trial cohort follow-up study. BMJ 2012;344:d7962.

46. Emmett SD, Schmitz J, Karna SL, et al. Early childhood undernutrition increases risk of hearing loss in young adulthood in rural Nepal. Am J Clin Nutr 2018. [Epub ahead of print].

47. Elmraid M, Mackenzie I, Fraser W, et al. Nutritional factors in the pathogenesis of ear disease in children: a systematic review. Ann Trop Paediatr 2009;29(2):85–99.

48. Curhan SG, Stankovic KM, Eavey RD, et al. Carotenoids, vitamin A, vitamin C, vitamin E, and folate and risk of self-reported hearing loss in women. Am J Clin Nutr 2015;102(5):1167–75.

49. Choudhury V, Amin SB, Agarwal A, et al. Latent iron deficiency at birth influences auditory neural maturation in late preterm and term infants. Am J Clin Nutr 2015;102(5):1030–4.

50. Melse A, Mackenzie I. Iodine deficiency, thyroid function and hearing deficit: a review. Nutr Res Rev 2013;26(2):110–7.

51. Martínez-Vega R, Garrido F, Partearroyo T, et al. Folic acid deficiency induces premature hearing loss through mechanisms involving cochlear oxidative stress and impairment of homocysteine metabolism. FASEB J 2015;29(2):418–32.

52. Nelson DI, Concha-Barrientos M, Driscoll T, et al. The global burden of selected occupational diseases and injury risks: methodology and summary. Am J Ind Med 2005;48(6):400–18.

53. Chadambuka A, Mususa F, Muteti S. Prevalence of noise induced hearing loss among employees at a mining industry in Zimbabwe. Afr Health Sci 2013;13(4):899–906.

54. Fechter LD. Promotion of noise-induced hearing loss by chemical contaminants. J Toxicol Environ Health A 2004;67(8–10):727–40.

55. Castellanos M-J, Fuente A. The adverse effects of heavy metals with and without noise exposure on the human peripheral and central auditory system: a literature review. Int J Environ Res Public Health 2016;13(12):1223.

56. Keppler H, Dhooge I, Maes L, et al. Short-term auditory effects of listening to an mp3 player. Arch Otolaryngol Head Neck Surg 2010;136(6):538–48.

57. Honeth L, Ström P, Ploner A, et al. Shooting history and presence of high-frequency hearing impairment in Swedish hunters: a cross-sectional internet-based observational study. Noise Health 2015;17(78):273–81.

58. Buszman E, Wrześniok D, Matusiński B. Ototoxic drugs. I. Aminoglycoside antibiotics. Wiad Lek 2003;56(5–6):254–9 [in Polish].
59. Mamun KZ, Tabassum S, Shears P, et al. A survey of antimicrobial prescribing and dispensing practices in rural Bangladesh. Mymensingh Med J 2006; 15(1):81–4.
60. Saunders JE, Greinwald JH, Vaz S, et al. Aminoglycoside ototoxicity in Nicaraguan children: patient risk factors and mitochondrial DNA results. Otolaryngol Head Neck Surg 2009;140(1):103–7.
61. Bortoli R, Santiago M. Chloroquine ototoxicity. Clin Rheumatol 2007;26(11): 1809–10.
62. Henry KR, Chole RA, McGinn MD, et al. Increased ototoxicity in both young and old mice. Arch Otolaryngol 1981;107(2):92–5.
63. Bongaarts J. Human population growth and the demographic transition. Philos Trans R Soc Lond B Biol Sci 2009;364(1532):2985–90.
64. Lin FR, Niparko JK, Ferrucci L. Hearing loss prevalence in the United States. Arch Intern Med 2011;171(20):1851–2.
65. Shangkuan W-C, Lin H-C, Shih C-P, et al. Increased long-term risk of hearing loss in patients with traumatic brain injury: a nationwide population-based study. Laryngoscope 2017;127(11):2627–35.
66. Staton CA, Msilanga D, Kiwango G, et al. A prospective registry evaluating the epidemiology and clinical care of traumatic brain injury patients presenting to a regional referral hospital in Moshi, Tanzania: challenges and the way forward. Int J Inj Contr Saf Promot 2017;24(1):69–77.
67. Alexander TH, Harris JP. Current epidemiology of Meniere's syndrome. Otolaryngol Clin North Am 2010;43(5):965–70.
68. Alexander TH, Harris JP. Incidence of sudden sensorineural hearing loss. Otol Neurotol 2013;34(9):1586–9.
69. Bovo R, Ciorba A, Martini A. The diagnosis of autoimmune inner ear disease: evidence and critical pitfalls. Eur Arch Otorhinolaryngol 2008;266(1):37.
70. World Health Organization (WHO). Deafness and hearing impairment. Available at: http://www.who.int/mediacentre/factsheets/fs300/en/. Accessed August 13, 2017.
71. Olusanya B, Neumann K, Saunders JE. The global burden of disabling hearing impairment: a call to action. Bull World Health Organ 2014;92(5):367–73.
72. Robertson SE, Featherstone DA, Gacic-Dobo M, et al. Rubella and congenital rubella syndrome: global update. Rev Panam Salud Publica 2003;14:306–15.
73. Mueller JE, Yaro S, Ouédraogo MS, et al. Pneumococci in the African Meningitis belt: meningitis incidence and carriage prevalence in children and adults. PLoS One 2012;7(12):e52464.
74. White KR. Reply to Olusanya et al: the role of the JCIH in the global expansion of newborn hearing screening. J Am Acad Audiol 2006;17:293–6.
75. Bilous J, Eggers R, Jarrett S, et al. A new global immunisation vision and strategy. Lancet 2006;367(9521):1464–6.
76. Wolfson L, Gasse F, Lee-Martin S-P, et al. Estimating the costs of achieving the WHO-UNICEF Global Immunization Vision and Strategy, 2006-2015. Bull World Health Organ 2008;86(1):27–39.
77. De La Sante O. Report of an informal consultation on strategies for prevention of hearing impairment from ototoxic drugs. Available at: http://www.who.int/pbd/deafness/ototoxic_drugs.pdf. Accessed August 13, 2017.
78. Chen Y, Huang W-G, Zha D-J, et al. Aspirin attenuates gentamicin ototoxicity: from the laboratory to the clinic. Hear Res 2007;226(1):178–82.

79. Harrison RV. Noise-induced hearing loss in children: a 'less than silent' environmental danger. Paediatr Child Health 2008;13(5):377–82.

80. Basner M, Babisch W, Davis A, et al. Auditory and non-auditory effects of noise on health. Lancet 2014;383(9925):1325–32.

81. National Conference of State Legislatures. Newborn hearing screening, state laws. Available at: http://www.ncsl.org/programs/health/ hear50.htm. Accessed August 13, 2017.

82. Olusanya BO, Swanepoel DW, Chapchap MJ, et al. Progress towards early detection services for infants with hearing loss in developing countries. BMC Health Serv Res 2007;7:14.

83. Elliott G, Smith AC, Bensink ME, et al. The feasibility of a community-based mobile telehealth screening service for aboriginal and Torres Strait Islander Children in Australia. Telemed J E Health 2010;16(9):950–6.

84. New Zealand Health Technology Assessment (NZHTA). Screening programmes for the detection of otitis media with effusion and conductive hearing loss in preschool and new entrant school children: a critical appraisal of the literature. Christchurch (New Zealand): NZHTA; 1998.

85. Brouwer MC, McIntyre P, Prasad K, et al. Corticosteroids for acute bacterial meningitis. Cochrane Database Syst Rev 2013;(6):CD004405.

86. Baltussen R, Li J, Wu LD, et al. Costs of screening children for hearing disorders and delivery of hearing aids in China. BMC Health Serv Res 2009;9(1):64.

87. World Health Organization (WHO). Newborn and infant hearing screening: current issues and guiding principles for action. Available at: http://www.who.int/ blindness/publications/Newborn_and_Infant_Hearing_Screening_Report.pdf. Accessed August 13, 2017.

88. Humes LE, Dubno JR, Gordon-Salant S, et al. Central presbycusis: a review and evaluation of the evidence. J Am Acad Audiol 2012;23(8):635–66.

89. Lin FR, Yaffe K, Xia J, et al. Hearing loss and cognitive decline among older adults. JAMA Intern Med 2013;173(4). https://doi.org/10.1001/jamainternmed. 2013.1868.

90. World Health Organization (WHO). Telemedicine: opportunities and developments in member states: report on the second global survey on eHealth. 2009. 2009. Available at: http://www.who.int/goe/publications/goe_telemedicine_ 2010.pdf. Accessed August 13, 2017.

91. Hassibian MR, Hassibian S. Telemedicine acceptance and implementation in developing countries: benefits, categories, and barriers. Razavi Int J Med 2016;4(3):e38332.

92. Kokesh J, Ferguson AS, Patricoski C. Telehealth in Alaska: delivery of health care services from a specialist's perspective. Int J Circumpolar Health 2004; 63(4):387–400.

93. Kokesh J, Ferguson AS, Patricoski C. The Alaska experience using store-and-forward telemedicine for ENT care in Alaska. Otolaryngol Clin North Am 2011; 44(6):1359–74.

94. Carroll M, Cullen T, Ferguson S, et al. Innovation in Indian Healthcare: using health information technology to achieve health equity for American Indian and Alaska Native Populations. Perspect Health Inf Manag 2011;8:1d.

95. Kokesh J, Ferguson AS, Patricoski C. Preoperative planning for ear surgery using store-and-forward telemedicine. Otolaryngol Head Neck Surg 2010;143(2): 253–7.

96. Kokesh J, Ferguson AS, Patricoski C, et al. Digital images for postsurgical follow-up of tympanostomy tubes in remote Alaska. Otolaryngol Head Neck Surg 2008;139(1):87–93.

97. Patricoski C, Kokesh J, Ferguson AS, et al. A comparison of in-person examination and video otoscope imaging for tympanostomy tube follow-up. Telemed J E Health 2003;9(4):331–44.

98. Swanepoel DW. Enhancing ear and hearing health access for children with technology and connectivity. Am J Audiol 2017;26(3S):426–9.

99. Boothroyd A. Adult aural rehabilitation: what is it and does it work? Trends Amplif 2007;11(2):63–71.

100. Abrams H, Chrisom TH, McArdle R. A cost-utility analysis of adult group audiological rehabilitation: are the benefits worth the cost? J Rehabil Res Dev 2002; 39(5):549–58.

101. Crowson M, Tucci DL. Mini review of the cost-effectiveness of unilateral osseointegrated implants in adults: possibly cost-effective for the correct indication. Audiol Neurootol 2016;21(2):69–71.

102. Wilson BS, Dorman MF. Cochlear implants: a remarkable past and a brilliant future. Hear Res 2008;242(1–2):3–21.

103. Gaylor JM, Raman G, Chung M, et al. Cochlear implantation in adults a systematic review and meta-analysis. JAMA Otolaryngol Head Neck Surg 2013;139(3): 265–72.

104. Crowson M, Chen JM, Tucci D. Provincial variation of cochlear implantation surgical volumes and cost in Canada. Otolaryngol Head Neck Surg 2017;156(1): 137–43.

105. Saunders JE, Barrs D, Gong W, et al. Cost effectiveness of childhood cochlear implantation and deaf education in Nicaragua: a disability adjusted life year model. Otol Neurotol 2015;36(8):1349–56.

106. Wong BYK, Hui Y, Au D, et al. Economic evaluation of cochlear implantation. Updates in cochlear implantation. Adv Otorhinolaryngol 2000;57:377–81.

107. Emmett SD, Tucci DL, Francis HW, et al. GDP matters: cost effectiveness of cochlear implantation and deaf education in Sub-Saharan Africa. Otol Neurotol 2015;36(8):1357–65 [Erratum appears in Otol Neurotol 2015;36(10):1765].

108. National Academies of Sciences Engineering and Medicine. Hearing health care for adults: priorities for improving access and affordability. Washington, DC: The National Academies Press; 2016.

109. Ruben RJ. Redefining the survival of the fittest: communication disorders in the 21st century. Laryngoscope 2000;110(2):241–5.

Management of Chronic Suppurative Otitis Media and Otosclerosis in Developing Countries

Adam Master, MD[a,b,c],*, Eric Wilkinson, MD[d],
Richard Wagner, MD[e]

KEYWORDS

- Cholesteatoma • Chronic ear disease • Chronic suppurative otitis media
- Otosclerosis • Stapedectomy

KEY POINTS

- Chronic suppurative otitis media is a major cause of acquired hearing loss in the developing world.
- Goals of treatment are to create a dry, safe ear and restore hearing with tympanic membrane repair.
- Health care workers should be trained to triage patients for surgery who do not respond to medical therapy, and identify complications of chronic ear disease that require urgent surgical care.
- Otosclerosis is prevalent and largely undertreated in the developing world.
- Surgeons on humanitarian missions should be prepared to address all complications of stapes surgery, and can expect to encounter a higher rate of obliterative otosclerosis.

INTRODUCTION

Chronic suppurative otitis media (CSOM) is a recurrent and persistent infectious process of the middle ear. In a subset of patients, the CSOM is associated with the

Disclosure Statement: The authors have nothing to disclose.
[a] House Ear Clinic, Department of Otolaryngology Head and Neck Surgery, Division of Otology, UCLA, 2300 West Third Street, Los Angeles, CA 90059, USA; [b] House Ear Clinic, Department of Otolaryngology Head and Neck Surgery, Division of Neurotology, UCLA, 2300 West Third Street, Los Angeles, CA 90059, USA; [c] House Ear Clinic, Department of Otolaryngology Head and Neck Surgery, Division of Skull Base Surgery, UCLA, 2300 West Third Street, Los Angeles, CA 90059, USA; [d] House Ear Clinic, 2300 West Third Street, Los Angeles, CA 90059, USA; [e] Global ENT Outreach, 1789 West Rebecca Drive, Coupeville, WA 98239, USA
* Corresponding author. House Ear Clinic, 2300 West Third Street, Los Angeles, CA 90059.
E-mail address: amaster@houseclinic.com

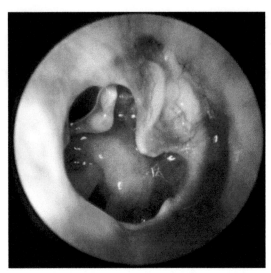

Fig. 1. Otoscopic view of a patient's right tympanic membrane perforation with discharge indicative of chronic ear disease. (*Courtesy of* Richard Wagner, MD, Coupeville, WA.)

presence of cholesteatoma. Both conditions are characterized by chronic aural drainage, hearing loss, and often tympanic membrane perforation (**Fig. 1**).

CSOM is a major cause of acquired hearing loss in the developing world and, if untreated, can lead to further morbidity and mortality in rare cases. Access to effective medical treatments, such as antibiotics, are often expensive and not widely available in most developing countries.[1] CSOM usually begins with one or more episode of acute otitis media, which eventually leads to a tympanic membrane perforation and a chronic infection. CSOM is defined by drainage lasting longer than 6 weeks, but may last for months or years despite treatment.[2]

Chronic Suppurative Otitis Media

Global incidence and prevalence

CSOM occurs on every continent, but occurs at a higher frequency among developing nations.[3,4] In the United States, CSOM occurs at a rate of less than 1%, whereas in many developing countries the higher rates of greater than 4% are observed.[5] However, the global prevalence of CSOM cannot be explained fully by the socioeconomic status of a particular country, with available prevalence data displaying heterogeneity within regions with similar socioeconomic status (**Fig. 2**).

In sub-Saharan Africa, there are a number of studies that examine the prevalence rates of CSOM in school children, with rates of chronic otitis media from 0.4% to 4.2%.[6,7] Studies from Thailand, Vietnam, Korea, and Malaysia showed a prevalence of CSOM from 0.9% to 4.7%. A recent study in India had a higher prevalence of 7.8%. Australian Aborigines were observed to have the highest prevalence rate with a range of 28% to 43%. Native Alaskans and Greenlanders also have high prevalence rates, ranging from 2% to 10%.[5] An Australian study of rates of hearing loss from CSOM varied among indigenous populations living in urban and rural settings. 0.7% of urban indigenous children had a 30-dB hearing loss or greater versus 20% of children in a Western Australian rural indigenous community.[8]

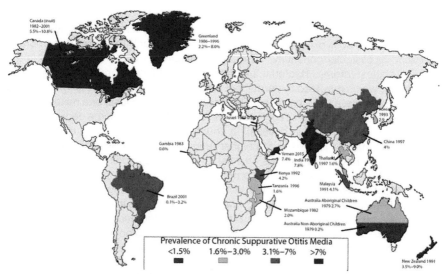

Fig. 2. Global prevalence of chronic suppurative otitis media. (*Adapted from* Campbell JL, Chapman MS, Dinulos JGH, et al. Leishmaniasis [Chapter 24]. In: Campbell JL, Chapman MS, Dinulos JGH, et al, editors. Skin disease: diagnosis and treatment. 3rd edition. Elsevier; 2011. p. 632–7; with permission; and *Data from* Acuin J. Chronic suppurative otitis media: burden of illness and management options. World Health Organization; 2004; and Muftah S, Mackenzie I, Faragher B, et al. Prevalence of chronic suppurative otitis media (CSOM) and associated hearing impairment among school-aged children in Yemen. Oman Med J 2015;30(5):358–65.)

CSOM development is multifactorial and may be related to a combination of risk factors such as:

- Crowded living conditions,
- Limited access to medical care including vaccinations,
- Inadequate antibiotic treatment,
- Exposure to tobacco smoke at home,
- History of bottle feeding, and
- Poor nutrition and hygiene.

The World Health Organization (WHO) considers a prevalence of CSOM of greater than 4% to be indicative of a "critical public health problem." Potentially addressing some of these correctable risk factors may improve rates of chronic ear disease. Establishing interventions at the primary care and community level can potentially impact the prevalence rates of CSOM. A study of Maori children in New Zealand supported this hypothesis when prevalence rates of CSOM were shown to decrease by one-half from 9% to 4% from 1978 to 1987, during which time efforts were made to improve treatment access and education.[9,10]

Community education and primary care interventions have also been shown to be effective for other global health issues.[11,12] In an effort to address such basic education issues, the WHO has developed *Primary Ear and Hearing Care Manuals* for basic, intermediate, and advanced levels of training.[13] The manual provides a tool detailing simple, effective methods for educating and motivating health care workers and community members to reduce the impact of ear and hearing disorders. The manual details all aspects of ear care, ranging from how to properly care and clean ears as well as the benefits of hearing aids.

Morbidity in chronic ear disease

Hearing loss occurs commonly in CSOM with a mild to moderate conductive hearing loss (CHL) in up to 50% of cases.[3] CHL may occur secondarily to tympanic membrane perforation or ossicular continuity. Ossicular continuity is much more frequent in the presence cholesteatoma. Bacterial infection of the middle ear may also spread to the inner ear, which may lead to permanent toxicity of cochlear hair cells The resulting hearing loss may be a CHL, permanent sensorineural hearing loss, or a mixed hearing loss. An estimated 534 million people are affected worldwide by some degree of hearing loss, of which 80% are in developing countries.[5] Higher rates of hearing loss in these regions may be related to the higher rates of CSOM in developing countries. For example, available hearing loss prevalence data of developing Pacific Island nations shows 3 to 5 times higher rate compared with other Australasian nations.[14]

Treatment for hearing loss is often very limited in developing countries. Hearing aids, are often not within the economic reach of most citizens in developing countries without the support of nonprofit organizations. Discounted hearing aids may be purchased by such nonprofit organizations through the International Humanitarian Hearing Aid Purchasing Program. Additionally, there is a dire need for hearing health professionals, including otologic surgeons. In a survey of Latin American countries examining the availability of hearing health providers, including otolaryngologists, audiologists, and speech pathologists, it was found that there was a scarcity of all 3 providers when compared with the United States.[15] Other studies examining Latin America concluded that hearing impairment is of low priority for most health systems and existing services are poor.[16,17] Similar, results were found in a survey of 18 African nations finding limited access to basic ear, nose, and throat (ENT) services, which are found primarily in major cities. Compared with the UK there was a shortage of 4755 ENTs, 20,856 audiologists, and 84,343 speech therapists in these African nations. Additionally, some countries have no ENT training programs, making it difficult to fill this large need.[18] There has been some recent success in establishing otologic health care in countries where such services were previously not available. In Malawi, a country of 18 million people, the lone otolaryngologist has established the first permanent ENT services and organized a team of clinical officers to provide services for 15,284 consults in 2012. Surgery was performed on 3% of these patients.[19,20]

Complications of chronic ear disease

Complications of CSOM can be subdivided based on the affected location. Complications are generally the result of spread of the infection from the middle ear and mastoid to adjacent sites. Spread may be intratremporal, extratemporal, or can even extend to involve intracranial structures. In the setting of mastoiditis, the highly pneumatized architecture of mastoid cortex can become "coalescent" secondary to bacterial erosion of the mastoid septae, which can be viewed on computed tomography (see **Fig. 2**). Bacteria can also access disseminate along veins or preformed pathways (eg, the labyrinth) to surrounding structures. Besides tympanic membrane perforation and hearing loss, the most common infectious complication of mastoiditis is the development of subperiosteal abscess from erosion through the temporal bone laterally (**Fig. 3**). The spread of otologic infections intracranially can be life threatening and should be treated as a medical emergency requiring urgent medical and surgical treatment.

Extracranial complications Mastoiditis accounts for 70% of extracranial complications, followed by facial nerve paralysis (12%), bezold abscess (10%), and labyrinthitis, sensorineural hearing loss, encephalocele, and petrous apicitis accounting for 2%

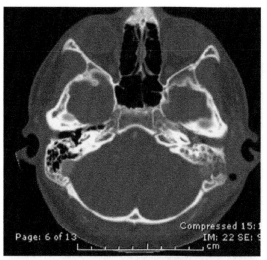

Fig. 3. Computed tomography image depicts a patient with a left-sided coalescent mastoid-itis with erosion of sigmoid sinus plate and extension into the subperiosteal area. (*Courtesy of* John L. Go, MD, Los Angeles, CA.)

or less.[21] Overall rates of mastoiditis in developed nations are low. Available data for Australia, the Netherlands, and Denmark show rates of mastoiditis at 2, 3.5, and 4.2 per 100,000 individuals, respectively.[22,23] Similar population-based data are not available for developing nations; however, a review of the available literature of all patients presenting to ENT facilities for all complaints in Zaire, Nigeria, Tanzania, Angola, and Sudan demonstrates rates of mastoiditis ranging from 1.5% to 5.0%.[6,24–27] In 1 study, 18% of patients with chronically draining ears presenting to an Ugandan ENT clinic had mastoiditis[28] (**Fig. 4**).

Intracranial complications Meningitis is the most common intracranial complication accounting for 51% of intracranial complications; brain abscesses are slightly less frequent occurring 42%, followed by sigmoid thrombosis at 19%.[23] Multiple intracranial complications may occur in 25% of cases reported from developing countries.[29] Prudent identification of patients with signs of intracranial disease is necessary, owing to the risk of death or permanent neurologic sequelae. A list of complications are presented in **Table 1**.

Global deaths from disease
Despite its generally benign nature, CSOM can lead to fatal complications in rare cases. In the preantibiotic era, mortality from complications of otitis media was common. In a 1935 review by Kafka[20] of 3225 cases of mastoiditis, the mortality rate was as 76.4%. The introduction of antibiotics has decreased but not eliminated the frequency and severity of complications. In a review of 93 Turkish patients with otitis media complications from 1990 to 1999, the mortality rates were 16.1% for all complications and 26.3% for patients with intracranial complications.[21] In a report of 155 cases of intracranial complications of otitis media from Brazil reveled that the majority were from CSOM (80%) rather than acute otitis media. The overall mortality rate in this study was 7.8%.[30] In another review of more than 24,000 patients from 1978 to 1990 with CSOM, intracranial complications occurred in 0.36% of the total with a mortality rate of 18.4%.[31] The WHO estimates that 28,000 deaths occurred

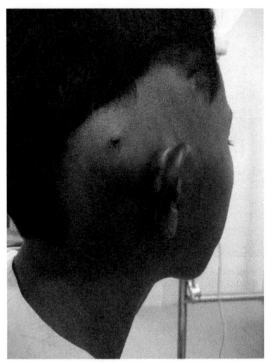

Fig. 4. Patient with marked postauricular erythema and swelling diagnostic of a subperios-teal abscess secondary to mastoiditis. (*Courtesy of* Richard Wagner, MD, Coupeville, WA.)

worldwide in 1990 as a result of complications of otitis media.[5] Current estimates of the Global Burden of Disease project indicate a revised global mortality from chronic otitis media to be 3194 deaths in 2015 (0.043 per 100,000).[5]

Global health management of chronic ear disease

The goal in managing patients with chronic ear disease is to create a dry, safe ear that no longer becomes infected and to establish a healed tympanic membrane to optimize hearing outcomes. There are 3 treatment options available for patients with chronically

Table 1 Potential intracranial complications			
Extracranial		**Intracranial**	
Extratemporal	**Intratemporal**	**Extradural**	**Intradural**
Postauricular abscess	Acute/chronic mastoiditis	Epidural abscess	Brain abscess
Bezold's abscess	Coalescent mastoiditis	Meningitis	Otitic hydrocephalus
Temporal root abscess	Labyrinthine fistula	Lateral sinus thrombosis	Subdural epyema
	Petrous apicitis		
	Facial nerve paralysis		
	Suppurative labyrinthitis		
	Encephalocele		

Data from Osma U, Cureoglu S, Hosoglu S. The complications of chronic otitis media: report of 93 cases. J Laryngol Otol 2000;114:97–100; and Kangsanarak J, Navacharoen N, Fooanant S, et al. Intracranial complications of suppurative otitis media: 13 years' experience. Am J Otol 1995;16:104–9.

draining ears: aural toilet, antibiotics, and surgery. Infection with cholesteatoma may be improved with antibiotics, but will recur unless definitive surgical management is pursued. Health care personnel must be able to determine the likelihood of patients responding to medical therapy, so as to prevent delays in surgical management.

Aural toilet
Aural toilet involves cleaning the ear canal using suction, forceps, basic irrigation, or other tools. It can be performed by family members or trained health care workers. The goal of aural toilet in theory is to reduce the bacterial load in the middle ear to help the immune system fight the infection and remove large collections of debris that may be a nidus for bacteria. Aural toilet is an important adjuvant to topical antibiotics; however, the benefit of aural toilet as a stand-alone treatment is questionable. A Cochrane review found there was no significant increase in resolution of infection or tympanic membrane healing with aural toilet alone compared with no treatment.[32]

Antibiotics
Antibiotics may be administered to the ear topically, orally, or parentally. Topical antibiotics have been proven to be more effective than parental and oral antibiotics in resolving drainage associated with chronic ear disease and are significantly less expense when compared with oral or parental antibiotics, thus, becoming the preferred choice.[33] Among topical antibiotics quinolones are more effective than other topical antibiotics.[34,35] Cost-effectiveness analysis demonstrates that topical antibiotics in combination with aural toilet is more cost effective compared with other treatments.[36] Based on this demonstrated efficacy and cost effectiveness, the current recommendations from the WHO include the combination of topical antibiotics and aural toilet as the medical treatment of choice for CSOM.

Surgery
Medical management is frequently only a temporizing measure in CSOM to decrease or temporarily stop aural discharge. Surgery including tympanomastoidectomy has the potential to remove diseased tissue and improve hearing deficits. Surgery is indicated in any patient with CSOM that does not respond to medical therapy or are unlikely to respond based on the severity of their disease. Patient with complications of CSOM require urgent surgical treatment. Unfortunately, the cost of surgery is prohibitive in most developing countries. The resources and equipment for performing otologic surgery is often relegated only to tertiary care referral centers in the major metropolitan areas. CSOM is often prevalent in the rural setting where the availability of surgical services is scarce. According to WHO estimates, 90% of patients with CSOM in Africa and 50% in South East Asia do not have access to surgical care.[5] These deficits in surgical care can be addressed by the training of surgeons in these regions, as well as providing the necessary infrastructure and equipment. The provision of care through humanitarian projects can be an important interim step toward this goal.

Establishing mobile clinics that bring surgeons with training in otologic surgery to areas of high need may be beneficial to provide short-term care, but is not sustainable if continuity of care is not fostered. The primary goal of humanitarian missions should be to help establish specialty otologic care among local providers in these communities so that the large need for otologic surgery can be met.

Various training initiatives have made attempts to develop clinical programs in developing countries. The "Oye Amigos" project performed 150 surgeries spanning 5 years with 15 four-day trips to Tepic Mexico in conjunction with the Mexican government.[37] Their tympanoplasty success rate improved from 41% to 74% after the first

2 years. They attributed this to the development of better patient education, and establishment of follow-up with local providers. Local providers may be able to see patients for follow-up visits, ear cleaning, and so on, and can assume eventual care of surgical patients.

One strategy that has been implemented in Malawi is to develop a certification program for midlevel providers to provide ENT services.[19] Before 2007, there were no ENT services in the country of 13 million people. With the establishment of an ENT Hospital in the capital, Blantyre, a 1.5-year certification program was developed in ENT and audiology for clinical officers. Clinical officers are not physicians, but have previously had 2 years of training and can act as midlevel providers. This local network of ENT care by clinical officers has vastly expanded the delivery of specialty care to the local districts. Establishing a permanent ENT service helps to improve international collaboration and allows opportunities for local physicians and providers to contribute to training and education. "Vertical" models such as these allow a limited number of physician otolaryngologists to establish a long lasting and self-sustaining model of health care in such low-resource settings.[38]

Choice of surgical technique

Generally in humanitarian circumstances, patients will not be seen on a regular basis and should be presumed to be noncompliant with follow-up visits or surgery. As such, most cases of humanitarian chronic ear surgery involving the mastoid should be canal wall down procedures. Staging chronic ear surgery in the humanitarian environment is rarely advisable. Patients must he presumed to be unreliable for follow-up, and procedures should be planned to be performed in 1 stage. Tympanoplasty may be sufficient for vast majority of patients with CSOM without cholesteatoma, but Horlbeck and colleagues[39] found that the addition of mastoidectomy (either intact canal wall or canal wall down) in draining ears resulted in better surgical outcomes. This result was presumed to be due to the removal of inflammatory tissue within the mastoid antrum.

OTOSCLEROSIS

Performing stapes surgery in a humanitarian setting or overseas requires that the surgeon be competent in the surgery, knowledgeable about potential surgical complications, and comfortable working in a new operative environment and with unfamiliar staff of different skill levels. When treating patients with otosclerosis in developing countries, the surgeon should:

- Be able to confirm the diagnosis with a tuning fork;
- Be able to treat obliterative otosclerosis without lasers; and
- Have an adequate supply of pistons in a variety of sizes.

Global Incidence

Although the true global incidence of otosclerosis is unknown, literature reviews demonstrate variation among races. Altman and associates[40] in 1967 compared the incidence of otosclerosis in the populations of whites and nonwhites. In the United States, the histologic incidence of otosclerosis is about 10% in the white population—even though, clinically, only 0.4% present with the characteristic CHL symptoms, with women having a slightly higher preponderance of clinical presentations than males.

Guild[41] performed histologic studies comparing blacks with Caucasians living in the United States and found the lower incidence of otosclerosis to be statistically insignificant, although the literature states that otosclerosis is about 7 times less frequent among blacks than among whites.

Although some reports suggest that otosclerosis is rare or nonexistent among Africans, these results may vary tremendously with the specific country. Otosclerosis has been described in indigenous blacks of South Africa [42] and otologists working on humanitarian projects with Global ENT Outreach have found otosclerosis to be relatively prevalent in Ethiopia (personal communication).

Likewise, there are variations in the prevalence of otosclerosis in the Americas. After examining 1258 temporal bones of Native Americans, Gregg and colleagues[43] found none with otosclerosis. Otosclerosis has been described in both Honduras and El Salvador, but personal experience of one of the authors suggests that it is more common in the El Salvador (personal communication). Honduras has a large multiracial population with some Caribbean heritage being relatively common, whereas El Salvador is isolated from the Caribbean. These racial differences may explain a potential difference in otosclerosis prevalence in these neighboring countries.

Many studies from Japan indicate that otosclerosis is more frequent among Japanese than among Africans, although less frequent than among Caucasians (**Table 2**).[44–50] Data on otosclerosis in the Chinese population are scarce. Choa[48] found that 100 of 1700 subjects from Hong Kong had otosclerosis.

There are no studies from the Pacific Basin other than that of Joseph and Frazer,[51] which studied the Japanese in Hawaii. The authors' experience in American Samoa, Fiji, and the Marshall Islands supports that otosclerosis is very rare in this region of the world. These studies are summarized in **Table 2**.

Audiologic Evaluation of Otosclerosis

In most developing countries, audiometric studies are performed by individuals who are often not adequately trained in audiology. Therefore, it is imperative to confirm the audiometric results by the use of tuning forks before a patient is operated on. This step will reduce the rate of false positives for CHL generated by improper masking or poor testing skills. The otologist should perform both Weber and Rinne testing with

Table 2
Global incidence study summary

Study	No. of Subjects	Race	Findings	Cases (%)
Gregg et al,[44] 1965	1258	American Indians	No cases of otosclerosis	0
Tato & Tato,[45] 1967	6000	South American Pure Indians	2 cases of otosclerosis	0.03
Tato & Tato,[45] 1967	4500	South American Mestizos	6 cases of otosclerosis	0.13
Goto & Takimoto,[46] 1967	1891	Japan	52 cases of otosclerosis	2.7
Takahara et al,[47] 1966	4082	Japan	21 cases of otosclerosis	0.5
Choa,[48] 1965	1700	Hong Kong	100 cases of otosclerosis	5.9
Nizar,[49] 1960	—	Indonesia	No cases of otosclerosis	—
Kapur & Patt,[50] 1966	414	East Indians	120 cases of otosclerosis	29

512-Hz tuning forks if the patient is seen in the clinic before surgery or in the surgical suite just before surgery.

Impedance audiometry, which includes both tympanometry and acoustic reflex testing, may not be available in developing countries. In cases of otosclerosis, especially when the disease is advanced, the height of the tympanometric peak decreases (type A_s). As the stapes becomes fixed, ipsilateral and contralateral acoustic reflexes are also affected. Normal reflexes in a patient with a normal otoscopic examination and CHL can signal the possibility of superior canal dehiscence syndrome. It is important for the surgeon working in developing countries to identify these cases without relying on routine computed tomography scans.

Hearing Aids

Hearing aids are an option for those with otosclerosis when surgical intervention is either unavailable or unwanted. However, the cost of the hearing aid, as well as the cost of the annual supply of batteries and servicing, may unrealistic for a patient living in a developing country where the annual income is less than $US2000.[52]

Role of Anesthesia in Stapes Surgery

Local anesthesia with sedation is well-suited to stapes surgery, especially in developing countries and in humanitarian work.[53] The advantages of local anesthesia and sedation enables one to make assessments in real time for immediate hearing improvement on insertion of the prosthesis, immediate vertigo potentially from an elongated prosthesis, and integrity of the facial nerve.

Although many drugs are available for sedation and analgesia, a combination of the following meets the requirements of safe anesthesia for surgery:

- Fentanyl 100 to 150 µg IV, once only.
- Versed 1 to 2 mg IV, once only.
- Lidocaine 1% to 2% with epinephrine, 1:30,000.
- Dexamethasone 12 mg IV, once only.

Surgery

Stapes surgery, whether it be stapedectomy or stapedotomy, is performed by surgeons with the same skill and planning in developing countries as in the surgeon's native setting. The surgeon should:

- Rule out other causes for CHL by reviewing the preselected cases;
- Confirm the CHL by testing with tuning forks;
- Ensure that all necessary instruments are available and ready;
- Prepare the prosthesis for implantation;
- Coordinate staff to assist with the surgery; and
- Counsel the anesthesiologist about the requirements for the surgery.

Prosthesis Selection

Many prostheses can be implanted in patients with otosclerosis to replace the diseased stapes and eliminate the CHL. In planning for stapes surgery overseas, it is helpful to:

- Use a prosthesis that can be cut to different piston lengths;
- Have a cutting block or similar tool; and
- Carry a few special pistons for incus necrosis.

One option is the titanium K-Pistons (4.5 mm length × 0.6 mm diameter; Kurz, Dusslingen, Germany) using the Fisch cutting block to cut the 4.5-mm pistons to any length between 3.5 and 4.5 mm.

Obliterative Otosclerosis

In developing countries, some otosclerosis patients may have CHL for years and even decades before undergoing surgery. Such patients are more likely to suffer from obliterative otosclerosis, in which the footplate can be thickened to between 0.5 and 2.0 mm. The incidence of obliterative otosclerosis among otosclerosis patients ranges from 7% to 11%.[54] Because of the higher percentage of obliterative cases, the surgeon should not rely on a hand drill or a pick to open or remove the footplate. Although these tools will suffice in many cases, a microdrill or a portable laser may be required for less traumatic removal of the superstructure and footplate fenestration.

REFERENCES

1. Cameron A, Ewen M, Ross-Degnan D, et al. Medicine prices, availability, and affordability in 36 developing and middle-income countries: a secondary analysis. Lancet 2009;373:240–9.
2. Kenna MA. Treatment of chronic suppurative otitis media. Otolaryngol Clin North Am 1994;27:457–72.
3. Monasta L, Ronfani L, Marchetti F, et al. Burden of disease caused by otitis media: systematic review and global estimates. PLoS one 2012;7:e36226.
4. Orji F. A survey of the burden of management of chronic suppurative otitis media in a developing country. Ann Med Health Sci Res 2013;3:598–601.
5. Acuin J. Chronic suppurative otitis media. Clin Evid 2004;(12):710–29.
6. Bastos I, Janzon L, Lundgren K, et al. Otitis media and hearing loss in children attending an ENT clinic in Luanda, Angola. Int J Pediatr Otorhinolaryngol 1990; 20:137–48.
7. Bastos I, Mallya J, Ingvarsson L, et al. Middle ear disease and hearing impairment in northern Tanzania. A prevalence study of schoolchildren in the Moshi and Monduli districts. Int J Pediatr Otorhinolaryngol 1995;32:1–12.
8. Watson DS, Clapin M. Ear health of aboriginal primary school children in the Eastern Goldfields Region of Western Australia. Aust J Public Health 1992;16: 26–30.
9. Smith AW. The World Health Organisation and the prevention of deafness and hearing impairment caused by noise. Noise Health 1998;1:6–12.
10. Giles M, Asher I. Prevalence and natural history of otitis media with perforation in Maori school children. J Laryngol Otol 1991;105:257–60.
11. Bhandari N, Bahl R, Mazumdar S, et al. Effect of community-based promotion of exclusive breastfeeding on diarrhoeal illness and growth: a cluster randomised controlled trial. Lancet 2003;361:1418–23.
12. Penny ME, Creed-Kanashiro HM, Robert RC, et al. Effectiveness of an educational intervention delivered through the health services to improve nutrition in young children: a cluster-randomised controlled trial. Lancet 2005;365:1863–72.
13. Nijmegen SH. Primary ear and hearing care training resource. Netherlands: World Health Organization; 2006.
14. Sanders M, Houghton N, Dewes O, et al. Estimated prevalence of hearing loss and provision of hearing services in Pacific Island nations. J Prim Health Care 2015;7:5–15.

15. Wagner R, Fagan J. Survey of otolaryngology services in Central America: need for a comprehensive intervention. Otolaryngol Head Neck Surg 2013;149:674–8.

16. Madriz JJ. Audiology in Latin America: hearing impairment, resources and services. Scand Audiol Suppl 2001;53:85–92.

17. Madriz JJ. Hearing impairment in Latin America: an inventory of limited options and resources. Audiology 2000;39:212–20.

18. Fagan JJ, Jacobs M. Survey of ENT services in Africa: need for a comprehensive intervention. Glob Health Action 2009;2:1932–9.

19. Mulwafu W, Nyirenda TE, Fagan JJ, et al. Initiating and developing clinical services, training and research in a low resource setting: the Malawi ENT experience. Trop Doct 2014;44:135–9.

20. Kafka MM. Mortality of mastoiditis and cerebral complications with review of 3225 cases of mastoiditis, with complications. Laryngoscope 1935;45:790–822.

21. Osma U, Cureoglu S, Hosoglu S. The complications of chronic otitis media: report of 93 cases. J Laryngol Otol 2000;114:97–100.

22. Bluestone CD. Clinical course, complications and sequelae of acute otitis media. Pediatr Infect Dis J 2000;19:S37–46.

23. O'Connor TE, Perry CF, Lannigan FJ. Complications of otitis media in Indigenous and non-Indigenous children. Med J Aust 2009;191:S60–4.

24. Mahoney JL. Mass management of otitis media in Zaire. Laryngoscope 1980;90:1200–8.

25. Okafor BC. The chronic discharging ear in Nigeria. J Laryngol Otol 1984;98:113–9.

26. Manni JJ, Lema PN. Otitis media in Dar es Salaam, Tanzania. J Laryngol Otol 1987;101:222–8.

27. Yagi HI. Chronic suppurative otitis media in Sudanese patients. East Afr Med J 1990;67:4–8.

28. Raikundalia KB. Analysis of suppurative otitis media in children: aetiology of non-suppurative otitis media. Med J Aust 1975;1:749–50.

29. Kangsanarak J, Fooanant S, Ruckphaopunt K, et al. Extracranial and intracranial complications of suppurative otitis media. Report of 102 cases. J Laryngol Otol 1993;107:999–1004.

30. Penido Nde O, Chandrasekhar SS, Borin A, et al. Complications of otitis media - a potentially lethal problem still present. Braz J Otorhinolaryngol 2016;82:253–62.

31. Kangsanarak J, Navacharoen N, Fooanant S, et al. Intracranial complications of suppurative otitis media: 13 years' experience. Am J Otol 1995;16:104–9.

32. Macfadyen CA, Acuin JM, Gamble C. Systemic antibiotics versus topical treatments for chronically discharging ears with underlying eardrum perforations. Cochrane Database Syst Rev 2006;(1):CD005608.

33. Browning GG, Picozzi GL, Calder IT, et al. Controlled trial of medical treatment of active chronic otitis media. Br Med J (Clin Res Ed) 1983;287:1024.

34. Esposito S, Noviello S, D'Errico G, et al. Topical ciprofloxacin vs intramuscular gentamicin for chronic otitis media. Arch Otolaryngol Head Neck Surg 1992;118:842–4.

35. Fradis M, Brodsky A, Ben-David J, et al. Chronic otitis media treated topically with ciprofloxacin or tobramycin. Arch Otolaryngol Head Neck Surg 1997;123:1057–60.

36. Baltussen R, Smith A. Cost-effectiveness of selected interventions for hearing impairment in Africa and Asia: a mathematical modelling approach. Int J Audiol 2009;48:144–58.

37. Barrs DM, Muller SP, Worrndell DB, et al. Results of a humanitarian otologic and audiologic project performed outside of the United States: lessons learned from the "Oye, Amigos!" project. Otolaryngol Head Neck Surg 2000;123:722–7.
38. Farmer PE, Kim JY. Surgery and global health: a view from beyond the OR. World J Surg 2008;32:533–6.
39. Horlbeck D, Boston M, Balough B, et al. Humanitarian otologic missions: long-term surgical results. Otolaryngol Head Neck Surg 2009;140:559–65.
40. Altmann F, Glasgold A, Macduff JP. The incidence of otosclerosis as related to race and sex. Ann Otol Rhinol Laryngol 1967;76:377–92.
41. Guild SR. Histologic otosclerosis. Ann Otol Rhinol Laryngol 1944;53:246–66.
42. Tshifularo MI, Joseph CA. Otosclerosis among South African indigenous blacks. East Afr Med J 2005;82:223–5.
43. Gregg JB, Holzhueter AM, Steele JP, et al. Some new evidence on the pathogenesis of otosclerosis. Laryngoscope 1965;75:1268–92.
44. Gregg JB, Steele JP, Holzhueter A. Roentgenographic evaluation of temporal bones from south Dakota Indian burials. Am J Phys Anthropol 1965;23:51–61.
45. Tato JM, Tato JM Jr. Otosclerosis and races. Ann Otol Rhinol Laryngol 1967;76: 1018–25.
46. Goto S, Takimoto I. Cases of otosclerosis in Japan. Jibiinkoka 1967;39:135–43 [in Japanese].
47. Takahara S, Saito R, Komoguchi H, et al. Statistical observations on otosclerosis. Nihon Jibiinkoka Gakkai Kaiho 1966;69:1547–54 [in Japanese].
48. Choa G. Some observations on otosclerosis amongst the Chinese in Hong Kong. Pac Med Surg 1965;73:8–11.
49. Nizar. The problem of otosclerosis in Indonesia. Madjalah Kedokt Indones 1960; 10:398–404 [in Indonesian].
50. Kapur YP, Patt AJ. Otosclerosis in South India. Acta Otolaryngol 1966;61:353–60.
51. Joseph RB, Frazer JP. Otosclerosis incidence in Caucasians and Japanese. Arch Otolaryngol 1964;80:256–62.
52. Available at: https://www.cia.gov/library/publications/the-world-factbook/rankorder/ 2004rank.html. Accessed July 16, 2017.
53. Bien A, WR, Wilkinson E. Local anesthesia in otologic surgery. Atlas of Otolaryngology Head and Neck Operative Surgery 2015.
54. Farrior B. Contraindications to the small hole stapedectomy. Ann Otol Rhinol Laryngol 1981;90:636–9.

An Evidence-Based Practical Approach to Pediatric Otolaryngology in the Developing World

Ryan H. Belcher, MD[a], David W. Molter, MD[b],
Steven L. Goudy, MD[c],*

KEYWORDS

- Pediatric otolaryngology • Global health • Developing country • Cleft lip
- Cleft palate • Foreign bodies • Hearing loss

KEY POINTS

- Involvement in global health and humanitarian efforts by US otolaryngologists has continued to increase the past 20 years, with pediatric otolaryngology surgical cases representing a large portion of cases.
- Otolaryngology services to underprivileged areas are limited by economic constraints, insufficient health budgets, poor infrastructure, and the minute amount of pediatric otolaryngology literature produced from developing countries.
- Literature from developing countries involve common pediatric otolaryngology diseases and surgical burdens including hearing loss, otitis media, adenotonsillectomies, tracheostomies, foreign body aspirations, and craniomaxillofacial surgeries including cleft lip and palate.
- When faced with poor resources and a unique disease burden, developing countries often must take an improvised strategy to treat pediatric otolaryngology disease processes.

INTRODUCTION

The care and management of pediatric otolaryngology diseases and congenital disorders plays a prominent role in humanitarian health care. A recent survey of American Academy of Otolaryngology – Head and Neck Surgery Foundation resident travel grants recipients from 2001 to 2015 showed that pediatric otolaryngology surgical

Disclosure Statement: The authors have nothing to disclose.
[a] Department of Otolaryngology–Head and Neck Surgery, Emory University, 550 Peachtree Street, MOT/Suite 1135, Atlanta, GA 30308, USA; [b] Otolaryngology–Head and Neck Surgery, Washington University School of Medicine, 660 South Euclid Avenue, Campus Box 8115, St Louis, MO 63110, USA; [c] Department of Otolaryngology–Head and Neck Surgery, Emory University, 2015 Uppergate Drive, Atlanta, GA 30322, USA
* Corresponding author.
E-mail address: Steven.goudy@emory.edu

Otolaryngol Clin N Am 51 (2018) 607–617
https://doi.org/10.1016/j.otc.2018.01.007
0030-6665/18/© 2018 Elsevier Inc. All rights reserved.

cases represented 51.9% of the surgeries performs. The only subspecialty of otolaryngology that had a higher distribution of surgical cases was facial plastics and reconstructive surgery at 63.5%, but many of these cases involved pediatric cleft lip and palate reconstruction.[1]

Despite humanitarian surgical groups, including otolaryngologists and trainees, traveling in record numbers to resource-limited areas, there remains a large burden of unmet need.[2] Otolaryngology services to underprivileged areas of the world are limited by economic constraints, insufficient health budgets, poor infrastructure, shortages of trained medical staff, and training programs.[3] In a survey of otolaryngology services in 18 countries in sub-Saharan Africa, even basic procedures such as myringotomy and tympanostomy tube insertion were not available to the majority of patients, which means it is possible that these patients could die from treatable ear infections.[4] A follow-up study reviewing data from 2009 to 2015 showed little progress in improving the availability of otolaryngologists, audiologists, and speech therapy services in these sub-Saharan Africa countries.[5]

Pediatric otolaryngology in the developing world is often faced with not only low resources, but with a different disease burden than the developed world. The increased prevalence of life-threatening infectious diseases such as human immunodeficiency virus (HIV) and tuberculosis have numerous otolaryngology manifestations. For example, these infectious pandemics are causing sensorineural hearing loss (SNHL) at an alarming rate, with 1 study showing up to 57% of patients treated for multidrug-resistant tuberculosis had SNHL, and up to 70% of patients treated for HIV had SNHL.[3]

The disparities in the developing world make it difficult to obtain quality data on the incidence or prevalence of pediatric otolaryngology diseases globally. Incidence or prevalence data presented in this article are mostly presented on a country-by-country basis, such as the prevalence of hearing loss (HL) in rural Nicaraguan children[6] or the geographic distribution of surgical burden of cleft lip and palate in Zimbabwe.[7] There is a meager amount of published information on otolaryngology that comes from the developing world. As would be expected, the little information that does come from developing areas of the world involve some of the most common pediatric otolaryngology diseases and surgical burdens including HL, otitis media (OM), adenotonsillectomies, airway obstruction requiring tracheostomy, foreign body (FB) aspiration, and craniomaxillofacial surgeries including cleft lip and palate. In this article, we discuss these issues and treatment strategies, and particularly how they differ in developed and developing countries. The challenges the developing world faces in treating pediatric otolaryngology disease process will be discussed as well as unique disease burdens they face.

COMMON PEDIATRIC OTOLARYNGOLOGY DISEASES
Pediatric Hearing Loss

Children with HL have been shown to be more likely to be unemployed as adults, have poorer academic achievement, and are less likely to finish secondary school.[8] Although this is devastating for children in both the developed and developing world, some studies have suggested that the burden, grave consequences, negative impact, and stigma of HL are more pronounced in developing countries, especially in the countries of South Asia, Asia Pacific, and sub-Saharan Africa.[9,10] According to the World Health Organization, there are 360 million people in the world with disabling HL with children comprising 32 million.[10] Developing countries comprise the majority of the global burden of HL, while also having a greater proportion of preventable HL causes. The World Health Organization reports that 75% of these hearing disorders in children age 15 and under are considered preventable in low- and middle-income countries as compared with 49% in high-income countries.[10] Some of these preventable causes include infections, such as cytomegalovirus (CMV), HIV, meningitis, measles, rubella, or chronic OM, as well as complications at the time of birth.

OM is considered the most common cause of conductive HL in children worldwide with developing countries carrying the greatest burden of OM among children, because it is a significant cause of disability and mortality.[11,12] There are several factors in developing countries that contribute to higher morbidity and mortality in children with OM that include crowding and poor hygiene, lack of access to adequate medical services, compromised immune systems from malnutrition, and early bacterial colonization of the nasopharynx.[11] Antimicrobial resistance is also a major problem in countries with higher density populations where antibiotics are easily obtained over the counter.[13]

HL is a known complication of children living with HIV and AIDS, which may result in conductive or SNHL.[14] Conductive HL in children with HIV/AIDS is mainly caused by OM. With the improved availability and the use of antiretroviral therapy (ART), lifespans of children affected by HIV/AIDS have been prolonged with some studies arguing this allows for more opportunities for acute and chronic OM infections,[15–17] whereas other studies have shown decreased episodes of OM in children with ART compared with those without ART.[18,19] SNHL in children with HIV/AIDS is mainly caused by opportunistic infections of the central nervous system, such as meningitis, encephalitis, or toxoplasmosis, affecting the auditory pathway in varying degrees. There is also a subset of patients with HIV/AIDS without opportunistic infection with high-frequency SNHL that is not fully understood.[16] There have been studies that show the potential for anti-HIV agents to be a source of ototoxicity, particularly an in vitro assessment that treated HEI-OC1 auditory cells with anti-HIV agents, alone and in combination, and found several of the agents to be toxic for these auditory cells.[20] Other studies have not been able to show conclusively that ART has ototoxic effects, specifically 1 study that did not show any differences in distortion product otoacoustic emissions between individuals taking and not taking ART, yet found significantly reduced distortion product otoacoustic emission magnitudes in the HIV-positive group compared with the HIV-negative controls. A possible explanation for this is a direct effect of HIV infections on the cochlea, although further studies are needed to elucidate this explanation.[21,22] The prevalence of HL among children with HIV/AIDS in the United States is 20%, whereas that in developing countries is much higher, with estimates as high as 42%.[14,16,23]

Congenital CMV (cCMV) infection is the most common cause of nonhereditary SNHL in childhood and has been found to be much more prevalent in developing countries.[24,25] The reported prevalence of cCMV in developing countries varies between countries, but is as high as 6% to 14% of life births. In contrast, most estimates from studies conducted in Europe, the United States, and Japan show their prevalence of cCMV to vary from 0.2% to 2.0%.[25–29] Approximately 10% to 15% of children with cCMV are symptomatic at birth, but the majority of children with cCMV are otherwise asymptomatic. Unfortunately, 7% to 15% of asymptomatic patients can develop late sequelae such as SNHL. Newborn hearing screens are almost nonexistent in the developing world so children with HL with other manifestations of cCMV are not diagnosed until school age at the earliest.[24]

Newborn hearing screens have become instrumental in the developed world in identifying children with HL before 6 months of age, because this time period is considered crucial for the normal acquisition of language.[30] Children identified with HL before

6 months of age and who are given appropriate support have shown to achieve better language outcomes than those identified after 6 months of age.[30,31] A study on the cost effectiveness of interventions for hearing impairment in sub-Saharan Africa and Southeast Asia shows through their mathematical modeling that screening of primary school children would lead to the treatment of a greater number children compared with the screening of secondary school children. It also showed that screening at the primary school level would yield greater health effects than screening at secondary school.[32] Despite the growing body of literature showing the major impact of newborn hearing screening has on the ability of children to obtain optimal speech and language outcomes, developing countries face many obstacles for the introduction of newborn hearing screening. For example, the costs associated with newborn hearing screening and follow-up services are generally beyond the capacity of many countries. Also, the burden presented by poverty, poor education, and other more life-threatening, fatal diseases also present a major impediment to the development of essential services for non–life-threatening conditions, such as HL.[30]

Tonsillectomies and Adenoidectomies

Adenotonsillectomy is one of the most frequently performed operations in children worldwide.[33] The indications for this surgery vary considerably between and even within countries. The absence of internationally accepted guidelines on indications plays an important role in this variability.[34] One study looked at the adenotonsillectomy rate for children aged 0-14 years of age between various developed countries in 1998 that showed dramatic variability between countries (19–118 per 100,000). This is summarized in **Fig. 1**.[34]

In the developed world, same-day discharge after adenotonsillectomy is a well-established practice, but in the developing world most of the patients after adeno-tonsillectomy are admitted for at least 24 hours of observation.[35,36] This procedure is also due to the fact that many patients in developing areas come from remote rural areas. For example, in Ethiopia with a population of more than 80 million citizens, 80% of the people live in rural settings.[37] Because these patients often live miles from paved roads or public transportation and these areas usually do not have skilled health care workers; any complication, especially bleeding, could turn into a life-threatening complication.[33,37] Owing to a lack of education, poor socioeconomic status, and a lack of physicians or skilled health care workers, many of these rural areas have local "traditional healers" that perform invasive procedures or

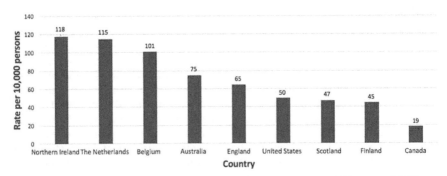

Fig. 1. Rates of tonsillectomies with or without adenoidectomy in children aged 0-14 years of age from various countries in 1998. Note the wide range of variability between countries. (*From* Van Den Akker EH, Hoes AW, Burton MJ, et al. Large international differences in (adeno)tonsillectomy rates. Clin Otolaryngol 2004;29;162; with permission.)

harmful health practices. In 1 study from Ethiopia, it is very common in Northern Ethiopia for "traditional healers" to perform tonsillectomies on children under 1 year of age by removing the tonsils with their index finger.[38]

The most common indications for adenotonsillectomy in the developing world are similar to the developed world such as recurrent infections and adenotonsillar hypertrophy, with obstructive symptoms as the most common reason for adenotonsillectomy.[39–42] Polysomnograms are not generally obtained in developing countries, owing to high costs, a lack of resources, and less trained medical staff.[27,37] Thus, the majority of obstructive sleep apnea is evaluated via history and physical examinations. Unfortunately, this means that the severity and degree of obstructive sleep apnea in these children is likely not accurately measured; several studies have shown that history and physical examinations do not associate with the gold standard for verifying obstructive sleep apnea, the overnight polysomnogram.[39,42,43]

All humanitarian surgical missions have multiple practical issues they must address. The issue of postoperative bleeding in tonsillectomy raises a particularly difficult issue because this complication can be both life threatening and delayed. Establishing a specific plan, which may include a relationship with a local general surgeon and possibly limiting travel, may be appropriate. In broader terms, teams may find the limitation on their surgeries may not be the technical rigor required for the procedure but for the postoperative period. Some procedures, such as cleft lip and palate repair, are particularly amenable to these "vertical" outreach trips as postoperative complications are in general not life threatening and can be corrected during subsequent visits.

Airway Obstructions/Tracheostomies

Tracheobronchial FB aspiration is a known life-threatening condition and requires urgent intervention. Children from 0 to 3 years of age are most susceptible to FB aspiration and a recent FB aspiration systematic review of 174 case series articles comparing high-income countries with low- to middle income countries showed that 75% of cases in high-income countries and 60% of cases in low- to middle-income countries were between 0 and 3 years of age.[44] It has been reported to be the fourth leading accidental cause of death in children under 3 years of age and the third leading cause of accidental death in children under 1 year of age.[45,46] Tracheal lacerations have been shown to be the most frequent complication in high-income nations, and pneumonia is the most often recorded complication in low-income countries.[44] Nuts, particularly peanuts, are the most commonly inhaled FB globally, but the assortment of FBs is wide and vary from country to country depending on diets and habits of the population.[44,47] In the United States, the incidence of pediatric FB aspiration resulting in airway obstruction is estimated at nearly 2.5 million per year with 350 to 2500 deaths per year; however, little is known about the incidence, morbidity, and mortality in developing countries.[48,49] Delay in diagnosis and treatment is an issue that plagues both developed and developing countries with dire consequences. The frequency of complications 2.5-fold higher in cases when bronchoscopy is delayed for at least 3 days.[44,50,51] Diagnostic delay is further aggravated in developing countries by lack of resources and awareness.

The gold standard for localization and removal of an aspirated FB is rigid ventilating bronchoscopy, with flexible bronchoscopy an acceptable alternative.[45,52] The introduction of the ventilating bronchoscope has reduced the mortality rate of FB aspiration from 24% to 2% and even less.[45] Unfortunately in low-resource settings, rigid bronchoscopy is often not available and transfer to tertiary centers with patients in respiratory distress is not possible.[48] A very large metaanalysis in 2013 on FB aspirations that specifically compared high-income with middle- to low-income countries reports the data are too poor in low- to middle-income countries to report rates of mortality.[38]

An unconventional, creative approach to managing FB aspirations has been described by using a flexible bronchoscopy to confirm the FB followed by tracheotomy with postural chest percussion with successful retrieval of the FB in 7 consecutive patients.[48] Postural percussion consists of lifting the child by the ankles and suspending the child upside down while performing chest percussion. This maneuver is performed until the FB is visible in the trachea and removed.[48]

Although quite rare, tracheostomies have been used for retrieval and complications from FB aspirations.[48,53] Tracheostomies have their own morbidity and mortality with the estimated tracheostomy related mortality rate of 0.5% to 2.0% in the United States.[54] Although it is difficult to quantify, it is presumed that this rate is much higher in developing countries.[55] As in the developed world, upper airway obstruction and long-term ventilation are the most common indications for tracheostomy in the developing world.[55–57] There are few data available regarding the role of tracheostomy in HIV-infected children, although 1 study from a low-to middle-income country showed that children with HIV presenting with croup have a significantly greater chance of requiring a tracheostomy and of delayed decannulation than that of non–HIV-infected children.[58] Although Groenendijk and colleagues[56] suggest that tracheostomy care at home is feasible under difficult socioeconomic circumstances with structured tracheostomy education and a caregiver training, resource-poor settings face steep challenges to discharge children with a tracheostomy home safely. In developing countries with unreliable electricity, parents of children with tracheostomies and who are discharged require a manual foot paddle-operated suction machine to help with their home tracheostomy care.[55]

Cleft Lip/Cleft Palate

Cleft lip and cleft palate are among the most common birth defects worldwide. The prevalence varies by ethnic and geographic ancestry with the highest rates in those children of Asian descent (**Table 1**). It is estimated that 70% of cases are nonsyndromic with cardiac, facial, and/or ocular defects being common in the remainder.[59,60] The etiology of cleft lip and cleft palate is multifactorial and consists of a mixture of genetics and environment, which can be influenced by cultural practices. Consanguineous marriages, maternal smoking, heavy drinking, folate deficiency, and teratogens, among other factors, play a role in the development of defects.[60] The significant impact that cleft lip and cleft palate has on most aspects of daily living, especially on communication, cannot be understated. Difficulty with speech intelligibility has a direct effect on education and employment.[61] It is estimated in the United States that there is a 75.6% unemployment rate for those with a significant speech

Table 1 Prevalence of cleft lip/palates in children by ethnic and geographic ancestry	
Ethnic/Geographic Descent	**Cleft Lip/Palate Prevalence**
Asian descent	1 in 500
European descent	1 in 1000
African descent	1 in 2500
United States	1 in 600–750

Data from Refs.[7,59,71]

disorder.[61] This impact is likely more significant in low- to middle-income countries. Muntz and Meier[61] discuss the financial impact of unrepaired cleft in the Philippines and stress that understanding the financial impact could influence governments of low- to middle-income countries to develop infrastructure for surgical care of the population with a cleft.

Parents who have children with craniofacial defects and the children themselves in the developing world face increased social rejection, isolation, teasing, and even infanticide.[62] In some societies, the parents are seen as being divinely punished for witchcraft, prostitution, adultery, and/or are cursed. The patients are regarded as evil spirits, ghomids, wizards, and sometimes not given names because they are not considered as "human beings"[62–64] In part owing to these social stigmas that patients and families face, there is an emphasis on early intervention for children in the developing world, although that is not always feasible owing to the socioeconomic and health disparities they face.[63] Data from large-volume, international surgical mission trips to Southeast Asia, India, and sub-Saharan Africa show that these patients often do not have their first reconstructive surgery until at least 2 or 3 years of age.[7,60,65] In the United States, it is generally accepted to repair a cleft lip around 2 to 4 months of age and cleft palate from 9 to 18 months of age.[66] Developing countries often do not have the resources for feeding adjuncts and milk substitutes for children with a cleft lip and cleft palate, resulting in a significantly slower weight gain in the first few months of life. Thus, some established craniofacial centers in those countries will repair their cleft lip and palate during a single-stage surgical procedure once child has reached a target weight of 3 kg. Alternatively, the procedures may be staged, but with both defects repaired by the age of 6 months of age.[64,67]

A large share of global humanitarian or mission-focused surgical service projects provide reconstructive surgery for cleft lip and cleft palate defects in resource-poor settings. There has been a large shift in the recent decades from an emphasis on the volume of cases to sustainability, education with host country providers, and health outcomes measurement of the entire care process.[1,7,68] The International Task Force on Volunteer Cleft Missions has commented that the major aims of any cleft mission are to provide high-quality surgical service, train local physicians and staff, develop and nurture fresh cleft programs, and make new colleagues.[54,69] It has been reported that there are increased complications and morbidity and mortality rates on these missions when compared with when the same procedures are conducted in the developed world.[68,70] This is thought to be due to difficulties in establishing a sterile field, genetic differences in the patient population, or poor wound healing secondary to malnutrition.[70]

REFERENCES

1. Jafari A, Tringale KR, Campbell BH, et al. Impact of humanitarian experiences on otolaryngology trainees: a follow-up study of travel grant recipients. Otolaryngol Head Neck Surg 2017;156(6):1084–7.

2. Volsky PG, Sinacori JT. Global health initiatives of US otolaryngology residency programs: 2011 global health initiatives survey results. Laryngoscope 2012; 122:2422–7.

3. Fagan JJ. Developing world ENT: a global responsibility. J Laryngol Otol 2012; 126:544–7.

4. Fagan JJ, Jacobs M. Survey of ENT services in Africa: need for a comprehensive intervention. Glob Health Action 2009;2:e1–7.

5. Mulwafu W, Ensink R, Kuper H, et al. Survey of ENT services in sub-Saharan Africa: little progress between 2009 and 2015. Glob Health Action 2017;10(1): 1289736.

6. Saunders JE, Vaz S, Greinwald JH, et al. Prevalence and etiology of hearing loss in rural Nicaraguan children. Laryngoscope 2007;117(3):387–98.

7. Tollefson TT, Shaye D, Durbin-Johnson B, et al. Cleft lip-cleft palate in Zimbabwe: estimating the distribution of the surgical burden of disease using geographic information systems. Laryngoscope 2015;125:S1–14.

8. Ruben R. Redefining the survival of the fittest: communication disorders in the 21st century. Laryngoscope 2000;110:241–5.

9. Adedeji TO, Tobih JE, Sogebi OA, et al. Management challenges of congenital & early onset childhood hearing loss in a sub-Saharan African country. Int J Pediatr Otorhinolaryngol 2015;79:1625–9.

10. World Health Organization. Deafness and hearing loss, fact sheet No. 300. 2017. Available at: http://www.who.int/mediacentre/factsheets/fs300/en/index.html. Accessed June 06, 2017.

11. Berman S. Otitis media in developing countries. Pediatrics 1995;96(1):126–31.

12. Kaspar A, Kei J, Driscoll C, et al. Overview of a public health approach to pediatric hearing impairment in the Pacific Islands. Int J Pediatr Otorhinolaryngol 2016;88:43–52.

13. DeAntonio R, Yarzabal JP, Cruz JP, et al. Epidemiology of otitis media in children from developing countries: a systematic review. Int J Pediatr Otorhinolaryngol 2016;85:65–74.

14. Torre P, Zeldow B, Hoffman HJ, et al. Hearing loss in perinatally HIV-infected and HIV-exposed but infected children and adolescents. Pediatr Infect Dis J 2012; 31(8):835–41.

15. Chao CK, Czechowicz JA, Messner AH, et al. High prevalence of hearing impairment in HIV-infected Peruvian children. Otolaryngol Head Neck Surg 2012; 146(2):259–65.

16. Christopher N, Edward T, Sabrina BK, et al. The prevalence of hearing impairment in the 6 months - 5 years HIV/AIDS-positive patients attending paediatric infectious disease clinic at Mulago Hospital. Int J Pediatr Otorhinolaryngol 2013;77: 262–5.

17. Jose R, Chandra S, Puttabuddi JH, et al. Prevalence of oral and systemic manifestations in pediatric HIV cohorts with and without drug therapy. Curr HIV Res 2013;11(6):498–505.

18. Miziara ID, Weber R, Araujo Filho BC, et al. Otitis media in Brazilian human immunodeficiency virus infected children undergoing antiretroviral therapy. J Laryngol Otol 2007;121(11):1048–54.

19. Sturt AS, Anglemyer AT, DuBray K, et al. Temporal trends in otolaryngologic findings among HIV-1-infected children in a population-based cohort. Pediatr Infect Dis J 2014;33(3):e76–80.

20. Thein P, Kallinec GM, Park C, et al. In vitro assessment of antiretroviral drugs demonstrates potential for ototoxicity. Hear Res 2014;310:27–35.

21. Maro II, Fellows AM, Clavier OH, et al. Auditory impairments in HIV-infected children. Ear Hear 2016;37(4):443–51.

22. Matas CG, Samelli AG, Magliaro FCL, et al. Audiological and electrophysiological alterations in HIV-infected individuals subjected or not to antiretroviral therapy. Braz J Otorhinolaryngol 2017. [Epub ahead of print].

23. Matas CG, Leite RA, Magliaro FCL, et al. Audiological and electrophysiological evaluation of children with acquired immunodeficiency syndrome (AIDS). Braz J Infect Dis 2006;10(4):264–8.
24. Goderis J, Leenheer ED, Smets K, et al. Hearing loss and congenital CMV infection: a systematic review. Pediatrics 2014;134(5):972–82.
25. Lanzieri TM, Dollard SC, Bialek SR, et al. Systematic review of the birth prevalence of congenital cytomegalovirus infection in developing countries. Int J Pediatr Otorhinolaryngol 2014;22:44–8.
26. Kenneson A, Cannon MJ. Review and meta-analysis of the epidemiology of congenital cytomegalovirus (CMV) infection. Rev Med Virol 2007;17:253–76.
27. Dollard SC, Grosse SD, Ross DS. New estimates of the prevalence of neurological and sensory sequelae and mortality associated with congenital cytomegalovirus infection. Rev Med Virol 2007;17:355–63.
28. Bello C, Whittle H. Cytomegalovirus infection in Gambian mothers and their babies. J Clin Pathol 1991;44:366–9.
29. Zhang XW, Li F, Yu WX, et al. Physical and intellectual development in children with asymptomatic congenital cytomegalovirus infection: a longitudinal cohort study in Qinba mountain area, China. J Clin Virol 2007;40:180–5.
30. Olusanya BO, Luxon LM, Wirz SL. Benefits and challenges of newborn hearing screening for developing countries. Int J Pediatr Otorhinolaryngol 2004;68(3): 287–305.
31. Yoshinaga-Itano C, Sedey AL, Coulter DK, et al. Language of early and later-identified children with hearing loss. Pediatrics 1998;102(5):1161–71.
32. Baltussen R, Smith A. Cost-effectiveness of selected interventions for hearing impairment in Africa and Asia: a mathematical modelling approach. Int J Audiol 2009;48:144–58.
33. Chussi DC, Poelman SW, Heerbeek NV. Guillotine vs. classic dissection adeno-tonsillectomy: what's the ideal technique for children in Tanzania? Int J Pediatr Otorhinolaryngol 2017. https://doi.org/10.1016/j.ijporl.2017.1007.1003.
34. Van Den Akker EH, Hoes AW, Burton MJ, et al. Large international differences in (adeno)tonsillectomy rates. Clin Otolaryngol 2004;29:161–4.
35. Riding K, Laird B, O'Connor G, et al. Daycare tonsillectomy and/or adenoidectomy at the British Columbia Children Hospital. J Otolaryngol 1991;20:35–42.
36. Masoom A, Akhtar S, Humayun HN, et al. Daycare adeno-tonsillectomy: is it safe in developing countries? J Pak Med Assoc 2012;62:458–60.
37. Isaacson G, Buchinsky FJ. More than a surgical mission–pediatric Otolaryngology in Ethiopia. Int J Pediatr Otorhinolaryngol 2011;75(8):1018–9.
38. Mitke YB. Bloody traditional procedures performed during infancy in the oropharyngeal area among HIV+ children: implication from the perspective of mother-to-child transmission of HIV. AIDS Behav 2010;14:1428–36.
39. Afolabi OA, Alabi BS, Ologe FE, et al. Parental satisfaction with post-adenotonsillectomy in the developing world. Int J Pediatr Otorhinolaryngol 2009;73(11):1516–9.
40. Orji FT, Ujunwa FA, Umedum NG, et al. The impact of adenotonsillectomy on pulmonary arterial pressure in West African children with adenotonsillar hypertrophy. Int J Pediatr Otorhinolaryngol 2017;92:151–5.
41. Antunes ML, Frazatto R, Macoto EK, et al. Adeno-tonsillectomy surgery in a joint aid effort: a feasible solution? Rev Bras Otorrinolaringol 2007;73(4):446–51.
42. Moghaddam YJ, Bavil SG, Abavisani K. Do pre-adenotonsillectomy echocardiographic findings change postoperatively in children with severe adenotonsillar hypertrophy. J Saudi Heart Assoc 2011;23:31–5.

43. Faramarzi A, Kadivar MR, Heydari ST, et al. Assessment of the consensus about tonsillectomy and/or adenoidectomy among pediatricians and otolaryngologists. Int J Pediatr Otorhinolaryngol 2010;74:133–6.

44. Foltran F, Ballali S, Rodriguez H, et al. Inhaled foreign bodies in children: a global perspective on their epidemiological, clinical, and preventive aspects. Pediatr Pulmonol 2013;48:344–51.

45. Hussain G, Iqbal M, Khan SA, et al. An experience of 42 cases of bronchoscopy at Saidu group of teaching hospitals, SWAT. J Ayub Med Coll Abbottabad 2006; 18(3):59–62.

46. Rovin JD, Rodger MB. Pediatric foreign body aspiration. Pediatr Rev 2000;21: 86–90.

47. Chinski A, Foltran F, Gregori D, et al. Foreign bodies in children: a comparison between Argentina and Europe. Int J Pediatr Otorhinolaryngol 2012;76S:S76–9.

48. Tamiru T, Gray PE, Pollock JD. An alternative method of management of pediatric airway foreign bodies in the absence of rigid bronchoscopy. Int J Pediatr Otorhinolaryngol 2013;77:480–2.

49. Karatzanis AD, Vardouniotis A, Moschandreas J, et al. The risk of foreign body aspiration in children can be reduced with proper education of the general population. Int J Pediatr Otorhinolaryngol 2007;71(2):311–5.

50. Huang Z, Liu D, Zhong J, et al. Delayed diagnosis and treatment of foreign body aspiration in China: the roles played by physician inexperience and lack of bronchoscopy facilities at local treatment center. Int J Pediatr Otorhinolaryngol 2013; 77:2019–22.

51. Lima JA, Fischer GB. Foreign body aspiration in children. Paediatr Respir Rev 2002;3(4):303–7.

52. Mohammad M, Saleem M, Mahseeri M, et al. Foreign body aspiration in children: a study of children who lived or died following aspiration. Int J Pediatr Otorhinolaryngol 2017;98:29–31.

53. Singh JK, Vasudevan V, Bharadwaj N, et al. Role of tracheostomy in the management of foreign body airway obstruction in children. Singapore Med J 2009;50: 871–4.

54. Rogers DJ, Collins C, Carroll R, et al. Operation airway: the first sustainable multidisciplinary, pediatric airway surgical mission. Ann Otol Rhinol Laryngol 2014; 123(10):726–33.

55. Zia S, Arshad M, Nazir Z, et al. Pediatric tracheostomy: complications and role of home care in a developing country. Pediatr Surg Int 2010;26(3):269–73.

56. Groenendijk I, Booth J, van Dijk M, et al. Paediatric tracheostomy and ventilation home care with challenging socio-economic circumstances in South Africa. Int J Pediatr Otorhinolaryngol 2016;84:161–5.

57. Sovtic A, Minic P, Vukcevic M, et al. Home mechanical ventilation in children is feasible in developing countries. Pediatr Int 2012;54:676–81.

58. Mulwafu WK, Argent AC, Prescott CAJ, et al. Tracheostomy in human immunodeficiency virus infected children at the Red Cross War Memorial Children's Hospital, Cape Town, South Africa. Int J Pediatr Otorhinolaryngol 2007;71:1125–8.

59. Kummet CM, Moreno LM, Wilcox AJ, et al. Passive smoke exposure as a risk factor for oral clefts - a large international population-based study. Am J Epidemiol 2016;183(9):834–41.

60. Brydon CA, Conway J, Kling R, et al. Cleft lip and/or palate: one organization's experience with more than a quarter million surgeries during the past decade. J Craniofac Surg 2014;25:1601–9.

61. Muntz HR, Meier JD. The financial impact of unrepaired cleft lip and palate in the Philippines. Int J Pediatr Otorhinolaryngol 2013;77:1925–8.
62. Fadeyibi IO, Coker OA, Zacchariah MP, et al. Psychosocial effects of cleft lip and palate on Nigerians: the Ikeja-Lagos experience. J Plast Surg Hand Surg 2012; 46:13–8.
63. Camille A, Evelyne AK, Martial AE, et al. Advantages of early management of facial clefts in Africa. Int J Pediatr Otorhinolaryngol 2014;78:504–6.
64. Van Lierde KM, Bettens K, Luyten A, et al. Speech characteristics in a Ugandan child with a rare paramedian craniofacial cleft: a case report. Int J Pediatr Otorhinolaryngol 2013;77:446–52.
65. Yao CA, Swanson J, Chanson D, et al. Barriers to reconstructive surgery in low- and middle-income countries: a cross-sectional study of 453 cleft lip and cleft palate patients in Vietnam. Plast Reconstr Surg 2016;138:887e–95e.
66. Goldstein JA, Brown BJ, Mason P, et al. Cleft care in international adoption. Plast Reconstr Surg 2014;134:1279–84.
67. Koskova O, Vokurkova J, Vokurka J, et al. Treatment outcome after neonatal cleft lip repair in 5-year-old children with unilateral cleft lip and palate. Int J Pediatr Otorhinolaryngol 2016;87:71–7.
68. Eberlin KR, Zaleski KL, Snyder HD, et al. Quality assurance guidelines for surgical outreach programs: a 20-year experience. Cleft Palate Craniofac J 2008;45:246–55.
69. Yeow VK, Lee ST, Lambrecht TJ, et al. International task force on volunteer cleft missions. J Craniofac Surg 2002;13(1):18–25.
70. Lee CCY, Jagtap RR, Deshpande GS. Longitudinal treatment of cleft lip and palate in developing countries: dentistry as part of a multidisciplinary endeavor. J Craniofac Surg 2014;25:1626–31.
71. Mossey PA, Little J, Munger RG, et al. Cleft lip and palate. Lancet 2009; 374(9703):1773–85.

Outcome of Head and Neck Squamous Cell Cancers in Low-Resource Settings
Challenges and Opportunities

Pankaj Chaturvedi, MS, FICS, MNAMS, Hitesh Singhavi, MDS,
Akshat Malik, MS, DNB, Deepa Nair, MS, DNB, DORL*

KEYWORDS

- Head and neck cancer • Developing countries • Tobacco • Challenges
- Opportunities • Resources

KEY POINTS

- Head and neck squamous cell carcinomas (HNSCCs) are among the most common cancers in several developing countries.
- There is wide disparity in care and control of HNSCC between developing and developed countries.
- Although they have a high burden of disease, developing countries often do not have the resources to adequately manage these cancers.

INTRODUCTION

Head and neck squamous cell cancers (HNSCCs) are the sixth most common cancers worldwide.[1] They are the most common cancer in some developing countries, especially in Southeast Asia.[2] In contrast, they constitute only 1% to 4% of all cancers in the Western world.[3] Worldwide, approximately 600,000 patients are diagnosed yearly with HNSCC, leading to 325,000 deaths every year. Although lesser developed regions accounted for 65% of newly diagnosed HNSCCs in 2012, they accounted for 75% of deaths.[4] Oral cavity cancers are the most common HNSCCs in Southeast Asia; whereas oropharyngeal cancers are relatively more common in the Western world.

Disclosure: The authors have nothing to disclose.
Department of Head & Neck Surgical Oncology, Tata Memorial Centre, Dr E Borges Marg, Parel, Mumbai 400012, India
* Corresponding author. Tata Memorial Centre, 1228, Homi Bhabha Block, Dr E Borges Marg, Parel, Mumbai 400012, India.
E-mail address: drdeepanair@hotmail.com

Otolaryngol Clin N Am 51 (2018) 619–629
https://doi.org/10.1016/j.otc.2018.01.008
0030-6665/18/© 2018 Elsevier Inc. All rights reserved.

ORAL CAVITY CANCERS

The oral cavity is one of the most common sites of HNSCCs.[5] Worldwide, among all HNSCCs, oral cavity squamous cell cancers (OCSCCs) have the highest incidence and mortality rate.[2,6] In 2012, annual estimated incidence and deaths due to OCSCC globally were approximately 300,000 and 150,000, respectively. An increase in incidence and mortality of OCSCCs is expected to take place globally. It is predicted that by 2020, these numbers will increase to 360,000 and 177,000 annually, respectively.[4]

Most OCSCC cases are reported in the low-income and middle-income nations. These countries contribute to 43% of the total number of newly diagnosed cases annually and about 50% of the global mortality.[4] These countries also have significant shortages of skilled labor, equipment, and health facilities.

Incidence

According to GLOBOCAN 2012, the global age-standardized incidence rate for OCSCC (per 100,000 per year) was 5.5. The incidence of OCSCC is quite variable around the world, with age-standardized rates ranging from as high as 30 to as low as 2. The highest incidence is found in Papua New Guinea, where incidence rates are 30 in men and 21 in women. Such a high incidence can be attributed to tobacco use (smoking and chewing), with alcohol and betel nut most common in this region.[7] For similar reasons, Southeast Asia also reports a high incidence of OCSCC, with incidence rates in men in these countries as follows: 15 in Sri Lanka, 15 in Bangladesh, 13 in Maldives, 11 in Pakistan, and 10 in India. Globally, India, with approximately 77,000 new OCSCC patients each year, ranks first in the total number of new cases registered annually. Hungary has the highest incidence rate[8] among all European countries. Other developed countries have lower incidence rates of OCSCCs in men: United States, 9; United Kingdom, 6; Germany, 10; and Japan, 4.

Incidence rates of OCSCC among women are almost similar with the highest incidence in Papua New Guinea with age-standardized rates of 21 followed by Melanesia with 16, Pakistan with 9, Sri Lanka with 6, and India with 4. Lower incidence rates in women are attributed to the lesser use of tobacco, betel nut, and alcohol. Even among women, the incidence is lower in developed countries such as the United States, United Kingdom, Germany, and Australia.[4]

Mortality

The mortality associated with OCSCCs strongly mirrors their incidence pattern. According to GLOBOCAN 2012, global age-standardized mortality rate for men is 2 (per 100,000 annually). Papua New Guinea not only has the highest incidence of OCSCC but also the highest mortality rate (16 per 100,000 annually). Similarly, other countries with high incidence that also report high mortality are: Melanesia, 11; Pakistan, 6; Bangladesh, 6; and India, 5. In contrast, the incidence, as well as the mortality rate, in developed nations is quite low. For example, the mortality rates in Germany, United Kingdom, United States, and Australia are all close to 1 per 100,000 annually. In developing nations such as India, 75% of OCSCC patients present at an advanced stage.[9] The mean age at presentation of HNSCCs is the fifth and early sixth decades in low-income economies, compared with the seventh and eighth decades in high-income populations.[10] **Fig. 1** shows the incidence and mortality of OCSCC in their increasing order of incidence, with a trend toward increased risk of OCSCC mortality as incidence increases.

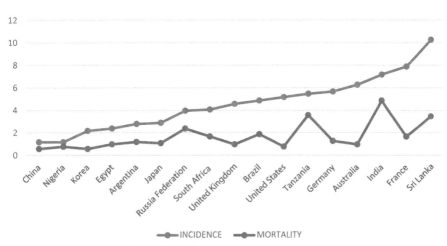

Fig. 1. Incidence and morality of oral cancer. (*Data from* Ferlay J, Soerjomataram I, Dikshit R, et al. Cancer incidence and mortality worldwide: sources, methods and major patterns in GLOBOCAN 2012. Int J Cancer 2015;136(5):E359–86.)

Etiologic Factors

OCSCC prevalence is higher in areas where tobacco is used in smokeless forms. Among African countries, Madagascar has the highest prevalence of smokeless tobacco use in men (23%), whereas Mauritania has highest prevalence (28%) in women. In Southeast Asia, the highest prevalence is seen in Myanmar, where about 50% of men consume some form of smokeless tobacco. A meta-analysis found that the overall risk ratio between smokeless tobacco and OCSCC was 1.8.[11,12] A study conducted by Sankaranarayanan and colleagues[13] in 1989 found an odds ratio (OR) of 4.3 in men for oral tongue and floor of mouth cancer with nasal snuff use, whereas the OR of gingival cancer with daily snuff use was 3.0.

Areca nut usage is associated with oral premalignant conditions such as oral submucous fibrosis, as well as OCSCC. This has predominantly been seen in South-Central and Southeast Asia, where areca nut usage is very common. The OCSCC, which develops in the presence of oral submucous fibrosis, is believed to be a clinico-pathologically distinct entity.[14]

Alcohol consumption has a higher risk for inciting development of floor of mouth cancer and tongue cancer.[15] According to the World Health Organization (WHO), Eastern Europe and the Americas have a higher per capita consumption of alcohol. Barring few exceptions, alcohol consumption in low-income and middle-income countries is generally relatively lower.[8]

The human papillomavirus (HPV) has been shown to be causally related to oropharyngeal cancers. HPV infection in the oropharynx tract generally occurs due to high-risk sexual behavior.[16] Association of HPV with OCSCC and larynx cancer has also been observed in several studies, although it is unclear whether HPV may be a true causative agent for a small minority of nonoropharynx mucosal squamous carcinomas of the head and neck. One study suggested that, although p16 expression was detected in 30% of tumors, only 4% of tumors were positive for HPV with in situ hybridization, thus concluding that OCSCC often overexpresses p16 but is rarely driven by HPV.[17] According to a systematic review analyzing 60 studies containing 5096 specimens in which polymerase chain reaction

(PCR)-based assay methods were used to detect HPV, the overall prevalence of HPV in HNSCCs was 26%, higher in oropharyngeal squamous cell cancer (36%) compared with OCSCC (24%) and laryngeal cancer (24%).[8] Studies from Taiwan, China, and Brazil have also observed an approximate 25% prevalence of HPV in OCSCCs.[18,19] However, it should be noted that many of the studies demonstrating higher rates of HPV prevalence in nonoropharynx subsites may be flawed with HPV detection methods with low sensitivity and specificity (eg, some PCR-based methods) and potential site misclassification of some tumors. According to a recent Union for International Cancer Control study, OCSCCs attributable to HPV was a meager 2.2%, whereas that for larynx was 2.4%.[20] Thus the aggregate of current available data and evidence suggest that contribution of HPV to oropharyngeal cancer is substantial but its influence as a causative agent for oral cavity cancer and laryngeal cancer is low.

Poor diet and nutrition have been found to contribute to the risk of developing oral premalignant lesions and OCSCC.[21–23] Chronic mucosal trauma, such as ill-fitting dentures,[24] sharp teeth, and poor oral hygiene, also can play a role in the causation of OCSCCs. These factors gain importance in patients from poor socioeconomic backgrounds who have poor oral hygiene and limited access to basic health care.

LARYNGEAL CANCER

Worldwide, around 138,102 new cases of laryngeal cancers are detected annually, resulting in 73,261 annual deaths. Cuba has the highest incidence rate (4.3 per 100,000) in the world. Incidence rates in developed countries are a little lower: United States, 0.7; United Kingdom, 1.9; Germany, 2.5; and Japan, 1.1. A higher incidence of laryngeal squamous carcinoma is reported in Southeast Asia, with incidence rates as follows: 1.7 in Sri Lanka, 2.7 in Bangladesh, 2.7 in Maldives, 2.9 in Pakistan, and 2.5 in India.[4]

Laryngeal cancers are potentially curable if detected early. Lasers have an important role in the treatment armamentarium of early laryngeal cancer. Unfortunately, their high costs and requirement of specialized training restrict their use in many developing countries. Total laryngectomy is the standard of care for advanced laryngeal cancers. However, postlaryngectomy voice rehabilitation is not universally practiced in low-resource settings. This is due to the high cost associated with tracheoesophageal prosthesis, equipment and maintenance, rendering this technology unsustainable in many centers. This has resulted in development of cheaper, low-cost prostheses in some lower resource settings. Unlike the scenario in developed countries where these prostheses are replaced frequently, the prostheses in developing countries may be changed less often and only when they start to malfunction.[25] Another example of a low-cost alternative is described in a review of literature on the international practice of laryngectomy rehabilitation intervention done in the developing country of South Africa. This review shows that a locally made cotton bib from simple cheap cotton eyelet fabric was superior to both commercially available heat and moisture exchanger filters and to commercially available cloth covers.[26]

PHARYNGEAL CANCER

The incidence rates of pharyngeal cancer in developed countries are 2.7 compared with 1.7 in developing countries.[4] Among the pharyngeal cancers, oropharyngeal cancers are by far the most common and account for the higher incidence of pharyngeal cancers in developed countries. Around 30% of oropharyngeal cancers (which mainly comprise the tonsils and base of tongue sites) are caused by HPV. The attributable fraction varies greatly worldwide, being highest in more developed countries (>40% in Europe, Northern America, Australia, New Zealand, Japan, and Republic of Korea) but much lower (<20%) and still uncertain in many developing countries.[20] An Indian study assessing the impact of tobacco on outcomes in patients with oropharyngeal cancer found a lower prevalence of p16 positivity (20%) and dual HPV and p16 positivity (38.8%) in the cohort. They did not find any significant difference in 5-year cause-specific survival between the p16-positive and p16-negative patients due to the existing high tobacco burden.[27] Treatment deintensification has been recommended for p16-positive oropharyngeal cancers.[28] Transoral robotic surgery is being used to treat oropharyngeal cancers amenable to it. However, due to the cost of the equipment and expertise required, the use of robotic surgery is limited to a few tertiary care centers in high-resource countries.

CHALLENGES

Developing countries face multiple challenges such as lack of awareness, illiteracy, reduced access to care, affordability of care, inadequately skilled labor, inadequate infrastructure, and sociocultural barriers. A study conducted in India found that there was a delay of about 7 months from the onset of symptoms to the initiation of definitive treatment in OCSCC patients.[29] This was in contrast to developed countries where such a delay ranged from 21 days to 3 months.[30] One of the most important deterrents to improvement in outcomes is a lack of accurate incidence and prevalence data for OCSCC. Most data comes from hospital-based registries, resulting in gross underreporting of disease. Thus, an important priority for developing countries is to establish population-based cancer registries. This will help bring the true disease burden to the forefront and aid health policymakers as they apportion health care funding.

Distribution of Research and Funding

Research funding is generally decided based on parameters such as incidence, mortality, finances, and years of life lost. Breast cancer, prostate cancer, and leukemia fall in the well-funded category, whereas oral cancer is generally underfunded. In the United States, in 2014, the incidence of oral cavity and pharyngeal cancer was almost similar to that of leukemia but research funding for leukemia was almost 20 times higher than for buccal cavity carcinoma. According to the National Institutes of Health, in fiscal year 2014, buccal cavity cancer and pharyngeal cancer were funded with $13 million compared with $236 million for leukemia.[31] However, research in a low-middle–income country such as India is more in accordance with the burden of the disease, making more funds available for HNSCCs. Indian researchers publish on OCSCCs 2.5 times more than the world average, which correlates well with the high incidence in India compared with the world average (6.10 vs 2.38).[32]

Percentage of Gross Domestic Product Used in the Health Sector

According to the WHO global health expenditure database, in developed countries, more than 10% of gross domestic product (GDP) is used in the health sector. The United States spends 17.8% of its GDP on health, compared with the United Kingdom, 9.1%; Australia, 9.4%; Russia, 17.8%; and France, 11.5%. In proportion, developing countries spend less on health care (India, 4.7%; China, 4.5%, Argentina, 4.8%; and Nigeria, 3.7%). Out-of-pocket expenditure refers to the percentage of private expenditure on health. It has been found to be high (up to 80%) in developing countries such as India (62.4%), Nigeria (71.7%), and Egypt (55.7%), whereas in developed countries it ranges from 30% to 50% (France, 29.1%; United States, 21.4%; and Germany, 57.3%).[33] A study by WHO showed that per-person health expenditure in developing countries such as India is about 54 dollars. In Russia, it is 525 dollars; in China, it is around 221 dollars. This expenditure on health is much less compared with the United States, United Kingdom, and France, where it is 8362, 3503, and 4691 dollars, respectively.[32] A prospective study was conducted to evaluate cancer economic burden on patients in India, from the time of diagnosis to completion of treatment. The average total cost of treatment to the patient was approximately 550 dollars, whereas the average monthly per person income for patients included in this study was about 28 dollars.[34]

Insurance

Recent studies suggest that patients without insurance are less likely to receive cancer screenings and are more likely to present with advanced disease and die from their cancers compared with those with insurance.[35,36] A study done on HNSCC patients in the United States showed that uninsured patients were at increased risk of death (hazard ratio 1.5). These patients presented with advanced stages of OCSCC (OR 1.95) and had a tendency of presenting with a higher number of positive neck nodes (OR 1.28).

Uneven Density of Skilled Labor

According to Global Health Observatory data,[37] the density of physicians in low-income and middle-income countries is less than 1 per 1000 individuals (India, 0.725; Egypt, 0.814; Nigeria, 0.4; and Sri Lanka, 0.7), whereas in high-income group countries it ranges from 2.5 to 3.5 (United States, 2.5; Germany, 3.9; France, 3.2; United Kingdom, 2.8; and Russia, 4.3). Low-income and low-middle–income group countries, which represent 48% of the global population, have only 20% of the health care workforce, or 19% of all surgeons, 15% of anesthesiologists, and 29% of obstetricians. Africa and Southeast Asia are particularly underserved. In terms of density, low-income countries have 0.7 health care providers per 1000 population compared with 5.5 in lower-middle–income countries, 22.6 in upper-middle–income countries, and 56.9 in high-income countries. In the developing countries, the specialists cater more to the urban population, whereas more than 60% of the population resides in the rural area.

Distribution of Radiotherapy and Chemotherapy

It is believed that most OCSCCs ($\leq$73%) end up requiring adjuvant radiotherapy.[38] The number of radiotherapy machines or centers in different countries varies. Developed countries generally have more than 5 machines per million population (United States, France, Germany, United Kingdom, Australia, and Japan). Developing countries have far fewer machines in comparison (China 1–3, India <1, Brazil 1–3, and Argentina 1–3 machines per million population).[39] Linear accelerator machines (linacs) are also differentially distributed. Germany has about 5121 linacs, the United States has 3416, France has 485, and the United Kingdom has 348. In comparison, developing countries have far fewer linacs: India, 232; Brazil, 290; Sri Lanka, 2; Egypt, 90; and Tanzania, 1. There is also a dearth of adequate numbers of radiation oncologists and physicists. In addition, there is a shortage of chemotherapy centers. Finally, the cost of most chemotherapeutic agents and supportive care is another barrier to effective cancer treatment.

Access and Affordability of Palliative Treatment

According to a study in the United States, the most common treatment of metastatic HNSCC patients was supportive care (90%) followed by surgery (49%), radiotherapy (42%), and chemotherapy (39%). The average 6-month incremental cost for palliative treatment was found to be $60,414.[28,40] Another study done in India found that in low-income settings, 81% patients opted for an inferior chemotherapy regimen if the cost incurred was greater than $1430.[29,41] Palliative chemotherapy commonly used for HNSCC consists of cetuximab or cisplatin and 5-FU (fluorouracil).[42] However, in lesser developed countries, HNSCCs are frequently seen in the lower socioeconomic strata of the society. Consequently, cetuximab-based combination chemotherapy is received by less than 1% of eligible patients.[43] Even conventional palliative chemotherapy is far too expensive for many patients. Oral metronomic chemotherapy has been tried as an alternative to conventional chemotherapy with encouraging results. These agents are significantly cheaper with lower toxicity profile, requiring less intensive supportive care, fewer admissions, and comparable oncologic outcomes. This is an area in which further studies are warranted.[41]

Access to New Technology

PET scan

PET–CT scans are considered the standard of care for workup of many locally advanced HNSCCs in high-resource environments.[44] However, in low-income and low-middle–income countries, the number of PET scan centers are scarce. According to a study in 2008, 22 functional PET-CT machines were available for patient use in India compared with about 2000 PET-CT scan machines in United States and 350 in Europe.[45,46] In India, the increase in numbers of PET machines over the last several years has not been commensurate with the increasing cancer burden in the country.

Sentinel node biopsy

Sentinel node biopsy (SNB) has been offered for clinicoradiologically N0 (node negative) patients as an alternative to elective neck dissection. On comparing the cost implications with quality of life in patients undergoing elective neck dissection versus SNB, it was found SNB was found to have the highest probability (66%) of being cost-effective at a willingness to pay of €80,000 per quality-of-life year.[47] However, this is not feasible in developing countries, where health care dollars are scarce and patients have low compliance with follow-up regimens. In such a scenario, doing an elective neck dissection is preferred.

Frozen section

Frozen section is widely used as a method to achieve oncologic safe margins during surgery. Frozen section adds to the surgical time, as well as to the overall cost of surgery and treatment. Also, advanced pathologic equipment for frozen section is not widely available in less developed countries. Indian studies have shown that gross surgical margins of 7 mm obviate frozen section and are oncologically safe.[48,49]

OPPORTUNITIES

Among HNSCCs, oral cavity cancers are ideal models for primary and secondary prevention. The oral cavity is easily visible for inspection and malignancies are often preceded by premalignant lesions such as leukoplakia or erythroplakia. Screening of high-risk population has been shown to be an advantage.[50] Health care professionals, including doctors, dentists, medical social workers, and other health care workers, should be sensitized to screen patients and educate them about harmful effects of tobacco, areca nuts, and alcohol. These are the ideal people to implement the awareness and screening programs with an emphasis on prevention. With better public awareness campaigns, the burden of the disease can decrease significantly. A good example of this is in India where second a Global Adult Tobacco Survey has resulted in a 6% drop in tobacco use.[51]

In most developing countries, health care is provided by the government, although government facilities are stressed with a high patient load. There is a definite need to increase GDP spending on health care and to focus on developing fully equipped oncology centers. There is a tremendous opportunity for low-cost innovation to make cancer care more affordable. An example is the development of indigenously designed radiotherapy machines such as Bhabhatron (Bhabha Atomic Research Centre, Department of Atomic Energy, India).[52] There have also been explorations of cheaper and yet effective chemotherapy regimens such as oral metronomic chemotherapy in the form of methotrexate and celecoxib.[41]

SUMMARY

HNSCCs remain common health problems in low-resource settings and are associated with a high mortality rate. There is need to establish more comprehensive affordable cancer facilities that comply with uniform treatment guidelines developed after regional consultation. To achieve this, the percentage of GDP allocated to health care should be increased in these environments, with a significant proportion directed toward cancer care and control. There is a need to accelerate primary prevention by creating awareness and educating people about the harmful effects of various carcinogens. Secondary prevention in the form of screening and early diagnosis needs to be implemented in community settings. Cost-effective therapies, further development of a skilled health care workforce, increased availability of radiotherapy machines, and cheaper chemotherapy drugs all remain high priorities.

REFERENCES

1. Parkin DM, Stjernswärd J, Muir CS. Estimates of the worldwide frequency of twelve major cancers. Bull World Health Organ 1984;62(2):163–82.
2. WHO | The global burden of disease: 2004 update [Internet]. WHO. Available at: http://www.who.int/healthinfo/global_burden_disease/2004_report_update/en/. Accessed September 2, 2017.
3. Bhurgri Y, Bhurgri A, Usman A, et al. Epidemiological review of head and neck cancers in Karachi. Asian Pac J Cancer Prev 2006;7(2):195–200.
4. Ferlay J, Soerjomataram I, Dikshit R, et al. Cancer incidence and mortality worldwide: sources, methods and major patterns in GLOBOCAN 2012: Globocan 2012. Int J Cancer 2015;136(5):E359–86.
5. Sankaranarayanan R, Masuyer E, Swaminathan R, et al. Head and neck cancer: a global perspective on epidemiology and prognosis. Anticancer Res 1998;18(6B):4779–86.

6. Joshi P, Dutta S, Chaturvedi P, et al. Head and neck cancers in developing countries. Rambam Maimonides Med J 2014;5(2):e0009. Available at: http://www.ncbi.nlm.nih.gov/pmc/articles/PMC4011474/.

7. Senn M, Baiwog F, Winmai J, et al. Betel nut chewing during pregnancy, Madang province, Papua New Guinea. Drug Alcohol Depend 2009;105(1–2):126–31.

8. Kreimer AR, Clifford GM, Boyle P, et al. Human papillomavirus types in head and neck squamous cell carcinomas worldwide: a systematic review. Cancer Epidemiol Biomarkers Prev 2005;14(2):467–75.

9. Patel UA, Lynn-Macrae A, Rosen F, et al. Advanced stage of head and neck cancer at a tertiary-care county hospital. Laryngoscope 2006;116(8):1473–7.

10. Sieczka E, Datta R, Singh A, et al. Cancer of the buccal mucosa: are margins and T-stage accurate predictors of local control? Am J Otolaryngol 2001;22(6):395–9.

11. Lee PN, Hamling J. Systematic review of the relation between smokeless tobacco and cancer in Europe and North America. BMC Med 2009;7:36.

12. Boffetta P, Hecht S, Gray N, et al. Smokeless tobacco and cancer. Lancet Oncol 2008;9(7):667–75.

13. Sankaranarayanan R, Duffy SW, Day NE, et al. A case-control investigation of cancer of the oral tongue and the floor of the mouth in southern India. Int J Cancer 1989;44(4):617–21.

14. Chaturvedi P, Vaishampayan SS, Nair S, et al. Oral squamous cell carcinoma arising in background of oral submucous fibrosis: a clinicopathologically distinct disease. Head Neck 2013;35(10):1404–9.

15. Jovanovic A, Schulten EAJM, Kostense PJ, et al. Tobacco and alcohol related to the anatomical site of oral squamous cell carcinoma. J Oral Pathol Med 1993;22(10):459–62.

16. Dahlstrom KR, Li G, Tortolero-Luna G, et al. Differences in history of sexual behavior between patients with oropharyngeal squamous cell carcinoma and patients with squamous cell carcinoma at other head and neck sites. Head Neck 2011;33(6):847–55.

17. Zafereo ME, Xu L, Dahlstrom KR, et al. Squamous cell carcinoma of the oral cavity often overexpresses p16 but is rarely driven by human papillomavirus. Oral Oncol 2016;56:47–53.

18. Luo C-W, Roan C-H, Liu C-J. Human papillomaviruses in oral squamous cell carcinoma and pre-cancerous lesions detected by PCR-based gene-chip array. Int J Oral Maxillofac Surg 2007;36(2):153–8.

19. Soares RC, Oliveira MC, Souza LB, et al. Human papillomavirus in oral squamous cells carcinoma in a population of 75 Brazilian patients. Am J Otolaryngol 2007;28(6):397–400.

20. de Martel C, Plummer M, Vignat J, et al. Worldwide burden of cancer attributable to HPV by site, country and HPV type. Int J Cancer 2017;141(4):664–70.

21. Doll R, Peto R. The causes of cancer: quantitative estimates of avoidable risks of cancer in the United States today. J Natl Cancer Inst 1981;66(6):1191–308.

22. Maher R, Aga P, Johnson NW, et al. Evaluation of multiple micronutrient supplementation in the management of oral submucous fibrosis in Karachi, Pakistan. Nutr Cancer 1997;27(1):41–7.

23. Nagao T, Ikeda N, Warnakulasuriya S, et al. Serum antioxidant micronutrients and the risk of oral leukoplakia among Japanese. Oral Oncol 2000;36(5):466–70.

24. Singhvi HR, Malik A, Chaturvedi P. The role of chronic mucosal trauma in oral cancer: a review of literature. Indian J Med Paediatr Oncol 2017;38(1):44.

25. Varghese BT, Mathew A, Sebastian S, et al. Objective and perceptual analysis of outcome of voice rehabilitation after laryngectomy in an Indian tertiary referral cancer centre. Indian J Otolaryngol Head Neck Surg 2013;65(1):150–4.

26. Fagan JJ, Lentin R, Oyarzabal MF, et al. Tracheoesophageal speech in a developing world community. Arch Otolaryngol Head Neck Surg 2002;128(1):50–3.

27. Murthy V, Swain M, Teni T, et al. Human papillomavirus/p16 positive head and neck cancer in India: prevalence, clinical impact, and influence of tobacco use. Indian J Cancer 2016;53(3):387–93.

28. O'Sullivan B, Huang SH, Perez-Ordonez B, et al. Outcomes of HPV-related oropharyngeal cancer patients treated by radiotherapy alone using altered fractionation. Radiother Oncol 2012;103(1):49–56.

29. Joshi P, Nair S, Chaturvedi P, et al. Delay in seeking specialized care for oral cancers: experience from a tertiary cancer center. Indian J Cancer 2014;51(2):95.

30. Hollows P, McAndrew PG, Perini MG. Delays in the referral and treatment of oral squamous cell carcinoma. Br Dent J 2000;188(5):262–5.

31. Carter AJ, Nguyen CN. A comparison of cancer burden and research spending reveals discrepancies in the distribution of research funding. BMC Public Health 2012;12:526.

32. Goss PE, Strasser-Weippl K, Lee-Bychkovsky BL, et al. Challenges to effective cancer control in China, India, and Russia. Lancet Oncol 2014;15(5):489–538.

33. Health expenditure, total (% of GDP) | Data [Internet]. Available at: http://data.worldbank.org/indicator/SH.XPD.TOTL.ZS. Accessed July 11, 2017.

34. Mohanti BK, Mukhopadhyay A, Das S, et al. Estimating the economic burden of cancer at a tertiary public hospital: a study at the All India Institute of Medical Sciences. Available at: https://www.isid.ac.in/~pu/dispapers/dp11-09.pdf. Accessed February 19, 2018.

35. Halpern MT, Ward EM, Pavluck AL, et al. Association of insurance status and ethnicity with cancer stage at diagnosis for 12 cancer sites: a retrospective analysis. Lancet Oncol 2008;9(3):222–31.

36. Ward E, Halpern M, Schrag N, et al. Association of insurance with cancer care utilization and outcomes. CA Cancer J Clin 2008;58(1):9–31.

37. Global health data repository: health workforce by category. Geneva (Switzerland): World Health Organisation; 2014. Available at: http://apps.who.int/gho/data/node.main.A1444. Accessed February 19, 2018.

38. Langendijk JA, de Jong MA, Leemans CR, et al. Postoperative radiotherapy in squamous cell carcinoma of the oral cavity: the importance of the overall treatment time. Int J Radiat Oncol Biol Phys 2003;57(3):693–700.

39. Available at: dirac.iaea.org. Accessed September 1, 2017.

40. Anuradha V, Anand BB, Suresh AVS, et al. Palliative chemotherapy in head and neck squamous cell cancer - what is best in Indian population? A time without symptoms, treatment toxicity score based study. Indian J Med Paediatr Oncol 2013;34(1):11–5.

41. Patil V, Joshi A, Noronha V, et al. Expectations and preferences for palliative chemotherapy in head and neck cancers patients. Oral Oncol 2016;63:10–5.

42. Vermorken JB, Mesia R, Rivera F, et al. Platinum-based chemotherapy plus cetuximab in head and neck cancer. N Engl J Med 2009. https://doi.org/10.1056/NEJMoa0802656. Available at: http://www.nejm.org/doi/full/10.1056/NEJMoa0802656. Accessed September 3, 2017.

43. Ignacio DN, Griffin JJ, Daniel MG, et al. An evaluation of treatment strategies for head and neck cancer in an African American population. West Indian Med J 2013;62(6):504–9.

44. Agrawal A, Rangarajan V. Appropriateness criteria of FDG PET/CT in oncology. Indian J Radiol Imaging 2015;25(2):88.
45. Buck AK, Herrmann K, Stargardt T, et al. Economic evaluation of PET and PET/CT in oncology: evidence and methodologic approaches. J Nucl Med Technol 2010; 38(1):6–17.
46. Rangarajan V, Purandare NC, Sharma AR, et al. PET/CT: current status in India. Indian J Radiol Imaging 2008;18(4):290–4.
47. Govers TM, Hannink G, Merkx MAW, et al. Sentinel node biopsy for squamous cell carcinoma of the oral cavity and oropharynx: a diagnostic meta-analysis. Oral Oncol 2013;49(8):726–32.
48. Mair M, Nair D, Nair S, et al. Intraoperative gross examination vs frozen section for achievement of adequate margin in oral cancer surgery. Oral Surg Oral Med Oral Pathol Oral Radiol 2017;123(5):544–9.
49. Chaturvedi P, Datta S, Nair S, et al. Gross examination by the surgeon as an alternative to frozen section for assessment of adequacy of surgical margin in head and neck squamous cell carcinoma. Head Neck 2014;36(4):557–63.
50. Sankaranarayanan R, Ramadas K, Thomas G, et al. Effect of screening on oral cancer mortality in Kerala, India: a cluster-randomised controlled trial. Lancet 2005;365(9475):1927–33.
51. Global Adult Tobacco Survey (GATS) 2016-17 revealed decreased prevalence of tobacco among young India [Internet]. Available at: http://www.biospectrumindia. com/news/59/9056/global-adult-tobacco-survey-gats-2016-17-revealed-decreased-prevalence-of-tobacco-among-young-india-.html. Accessed July 29, 2017.
52. PM Modi hands over Bhabhatron machine to Mongolia for cancer treatment [Internet]. Firstpost. 2015. Available at: http://www.firstpost.com/world/pm-modi-hands-bhabhatron-machine-mongolia-cancer-treatment-2248696.html. Accessed July 29, 2017.

Thyroid Disease Around the World

Anastasios Maniakas, MD[a], Louise Davies, MD, MS[b], Mark E. Zafereo, MD[c],*

KEYWORDS

- Thyroid disease • Thyroid cancer • Iodine deficiency • Thyroid surgery
- Developed world • Developing world • Low-resource setting

KEY POINTS

- Iodine deficiency is one of the world's most prevalent nutrient deficiencies, heavily associated with the development of an epidemic of goitrous thyroid glands.
- Thyroid cancer rates are significantly on the rise although overall thyroid cancer–associated mortality is fortunately not following suit; therefore, one must be cautious of potential over-screening and overdiagnosis.
- Thyroid surgery in the developing world can vary from that performed in the developed world and should be performed in accordance with the resource setting and patient compliance.
- With the increase in thyroid cancer incidence, the economic burden of the disease will continue to increase. Efficiency and selective treatment will be key in the future.

Thyroid disease will affect approximately 1 in 20 Americans in their lifetime, with women being approximately 7-fold more likely to be affected.[1] In fact, 1 in 8 women in the United States will develop a thyroid disorder at some point during their lifetime.[1] The most common form of thyroid disorder remains thyroid goiter, whereas thyroid cancer is the most common endocrine neoplasia and represents approximately 1.5% to 2.1% of all cancers diagnosed annually worldwide.[2,3] As such, this article focuses on 2 of the most clinically important subgroups of thyroid disease: iodine deficiency and thyroid goiter, and thyroid cancer.

IODINE DEFICIENCY AND GOITROUS THYROID

Iodine deficiency is one of the world's most prevalent yet preventable nutrient deficiencies, affecting an estimated 35% to 40% of the world's population,[4] and is

---

Disclosure Statement: The authors have nothing to disclose.
[a] Division of Otolaryngology–Head and Neck Surgery, Department of Surgery, Université de Montréal, 5775 boul. Léger, Montréal, Québec, Canada H1G 1K7; [b] Department of Surgery-Otolaryngology, Geisel School of Medicine at Dartmouth, 1 Rope Ferry Road, Hanover, NH 03755, USA; [c] Department of Head and Neck Surgery, Division of Surgery, The University of Texas MD Anderson Cancer Center, 1515 Holcombe Boulevard, Unit 1445, Houston, TX 77030, USA
* Corresponding author.
E-mail address: mzafereo@mdanderson.org

Otolaryngol Clin N Am 51 (2018) 631–642
https://doi.org/10.1016/j.otc.2018.01.014
0030-6665/18/© 2018 Elsevier Inc. All rights reserved.
oto.theclinics.com

considered a public health problem in almost 50 countries.[5] Other than the development of goitrous thyroid glands, iodine deficiency causes a wide spectrum of disorders, such as mental retardation, stunted growth, brain damage, congenital defects, and stillbirth, among others. Death directly secondary to iodine deficiency is not common (1 per one million people per year); however, it is principally found in the poorly developed countries of Africa and Central and Southeast Asia (**Fig. 1**).[6] Furthermore, iodine deficiency has been shown to be associated with higher rates of follicular thyroid carcinoma as well as poorly differentiated and anaplastic carcinoma.[7] The International Child Development Steering Group identified iodine deficiency as one of the 4 key global risk factors for impaired child development, whereby the need for intervention is urgent.[8] Salt iodization is the most cost-effective way of delivering iodine in deficient populations. It is clear in the World Health Organization's recent statement that salt iodization is imperative and clearly demonstrates that when implemented, it significantly reduces the risk and prevalence of goiter as well as other iodine deficiency disorders.[9] Furthermore, studies have shown a shift in the subtypes of thyroid cancer, with higher papillary to follicular thyroid carcinoma ratios and a decrease in the percentage of anaplastic thyroid carcinomas, in regions where salt iodization was introduced or increased.[10]

Thyroid goiter is primarily benign and affects approximately 7% of the worldwide population. Goiter is, however, associated with thyroid cancer. Thyroid cancer has been reportedly found in 10% to 15% of goiters[11,12] and as high as in 20% in endemic multinodular goiter regions.[13,14] Furthermore, in poor rural areas in Sub-Saharan Africa, where cassava is commonly eaten, linamarin (a cyanogenic glucoside) significantly increases the severity of goiter endemia.[15] Interestingly, although thyroid cancer rates are generally higher in women, when it comes to goiter-associated incidental thyroid cancer, one study has suggested that male sex and younger age may be risk factors.[16]

Goiters can be nontoxic or toxic and may induce compressive symptoms and cosmetic deformities. Although globally goiters are principally secondary to iodine deficiency, in countries where iodine deficiency is not a major factor, multinodular thyroid disease, chronic autoimmune thyroiditis, and Grave disease are common causes

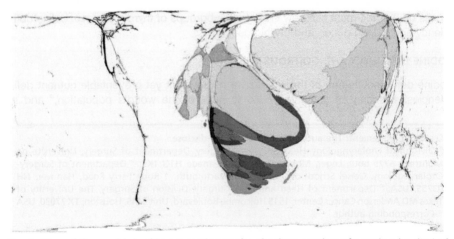

Fig. 1. Map of the world sized in proportion to the absolute number of people who died of iodine deficiency in 1 year. (*From* Worldmapper. Map number 415: iodine deficiency deaths. Available at: http://www.worldmapper.org/. Accessed June 20, 2017; with permission.)

of goiter.[12] Goiters associated with iodine deficiency are often treated with iodine. However, when goiters do not regress or when they show compressive symptoms as can be seen with large multinodular goiter, surgical removal of all or part of the thyroid gland may be considered.

Options for thyroid goiter surgery include thyroid lobectomy (dominant lobe), subtotal thyroidectomy, and total thyroidectomy. Benefits of total thyroidectomy include complete goiter removal and decreased recurrence risk. If a subtotal procedure is performed, then the patient, especially of young age, will be at risk for goiter recurrence over time (often within 10 years).[17] However, patients who undergo a total thyroidectomy, especially in a low-resource setting, have increased surgical risks related to recurrent laryngeal nerve injury, hypoparathyroidism, and hypothyroidism. In regions where economic and medical structural resources are lacking, some patients may have limited access to long-term thyroid hormone, making them susceptible to the morbidity and mortality related to hypothyroidism.

It has been suggested that excision of dominant thyroid nodules, lobectomy, or subtotal thyroidectomy may be a viable option for the elderly in an attempt to spare them of the excess morbidity associated with a total thyroidectomy,[18] as even temporary hypoparathyroidism can be a potentially deadly complication in a setting where a patient's access to intravenous/oral calcium and synthetic vitamin D are limited. In addition, patients who undergo total thyroidectomy are required to remain on lifelong thyroid replacement hormone medication, whereas only approximately 15% to 25% of patients undergoing thyroid lobectomy may require some degree of thyroid hormone supplementation in order to maintain normal thyroid hormone function.[19,20] In the case of goiters, even with subtotal thyroidectomy, remnant thyroid parenchyma, which is often diseased and nodular, may result in postoperative hypothyroidism subsequently needing hormone replacement.[21,22]

THYROID CANCER

Thyroid cancer can be generally subdivided into well-differentiated and non-differentiated thyroid cancer, with the well-differentiated papillary subtype being the most common. More specifically, papillary, follicular, and Hurthle cell carcinoma make up about 95% of all thyroid cancers. Since 1973, the annual incidence of thyroid cancer in the United States has increased more than 500%,[23] with increases seen across all tumor sizes (**Fig. 2**).[24] Overall, thyroid cancer incidence has increased across all continents except Africa, likely because of lower rates of access to ultrasound and cross-sectional imaging.[25]

In fact, incidence rates are more than 2-fold higher in high-income countries as compared with low-/middle-income countries for both women and men,[26] and similarly when one compares developed versus developing countries (**Fig. 3**).[27] This socioeconomic discrepancy is likely due to the immediate and abundant access to health care in high-income countries. This phenomenon has been reported even within high-income countries, such as the United States, where 2 neighboring counties may have significantly different papillary cancer incidence rates, with the difference directly correlating with respective patient mean household incomes and education level.[28] As such, because of higher mean household incomes and education, these patients tend to have increased access to health care. With computed tomography scans able to detect nodules as small as 0.2 cm, along with the widespread use of ultrasonography, MRI, PET, and cardiac nuclear medicine scans for nonthyroid imaging, overdetection and overinvestigation of small subclinical nodules have become common in developed countries. These small, incidentally discovered

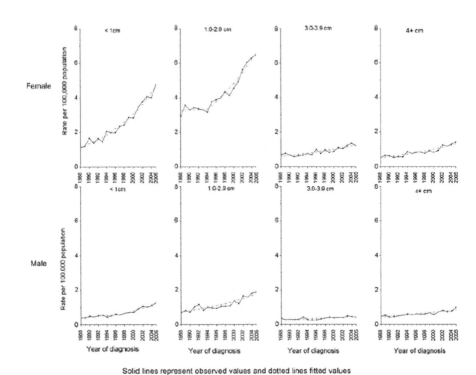

Solid lines represent observed values and dotted lines fitted values

Fig. 2. Increase in thyroid cancer incidence rates from 1988 through 2005 according to tumor size (<1 cm, 1–2.9 cm, 3–3.9 cm, and ≥4 cm). (*From* Chen AY, Jemal A, Ward EM. Increasing incidence of differentiated thyroid cancer in the United States, 1988-2005. Cancer 2009;115:3806; with permission.)

thyroid nodules, often termed "incidentalomas," are benign in their vast majority. When malignant, these incidentalomas are principally of the papillary subtype and account for much of the increase of thyroid cancer incidence in the past decade[29] (**Figs. 4** and **5**).[26,30] Overall, if current trends in thyroid cancer continue, it is estimated that thyroid cancer may be the fourth most common cancer in the United States by 2030 (**Fig. 6**).[31] In South Korea, where cancer screening was implemented in 1999, the rate of thyroid cancer diagnosis increased 15-fold, with mortalities remaining unchanged, making it the most common type of cancer in the country in 2011.[32] However, following reforms in 2014 to prevent the overdiagnosis of thyroid cancer, there was a rapid 30% reduction in the rates of thyroid surgery resulting directly from less screening.[33]

In the United States, a recent study demonstrated that although the overall increase in thyroid cancer rate was likely attributable to overdiagnosis, incidence rates and mortality for patients presenting with distant disease at the time of diagnosis were both increasing. The investigators suggested that this finding was more consistent with a true increase in thyroid cancer than overdiagnosis[34] and recommended research directed at potential reasons for the true increase as well as efforts to improve treatment of metastatic disease.[35]

Other than inherited risk factors such as with multiple endocrine neoplasia type 2, known external risk factors for thyroid cancer include radiation exposure before age 20 (eg, through medical imaging, therapeutic radiation, natural radiation, or nuclear

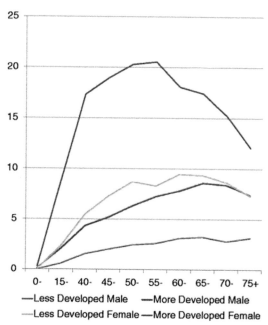

Fig. 3. Incidence rates (per 100,000 per year) in male and female patients in more or less developed countries according to age. (*From* Magrath I, Epelman S. Cancer in adolescents and young adults in countries with limited resources. Curr Oncol Rep 2013;15:341; with permission.)

accidents) and potentially an iodine-deficient diet, with both of these factors having long-standing effects, especially if the individual is exposed at a very young age.[36,37] Moreover, studies from the Chernobyl accident suggest that iodine deficiency in radiation-exposed children conferred an additional 2 to 3 times greater risk of developing thyroid cancer when compared with children who were iodine sufficient at the time of their exposure.[10] Presently, thyroid cancer is the most common cancer in Americans aged 16 to 33 years,[38] and although mortalities in children and young adults are not greater than they are for adults, survivors have to live with side effects and complications of such interventions for decades following their treatment.

Even though the incidence of thyroid cancer continues to increase, mortalities have fortunately remained steady or declined.[26,39] This decline may be due to the earlier diagnosis of thyroid cancer secondary to fortuitous early detection along with quick therapeutic intervention. Although evidence is limited, it has been hypothesized that as the rates of iodine deficiency decrease, so do the rates of iodine deficient–associated thyroid cancer subtypes, that is, follicular and anaplastic cancers, which are often more aggressive than papillary cancers.[10] Zimmerman and Galetti[10] further demonstrated a weak but statistically significant correlation between a greater increase in iodine intake and a greater decrease in thyroid cancer mortality, however, only for women. Although they were not evaluating thyroid cancer mortality, a similar variation was reported by Woodruff and colleagues[40] in a study where the change in thyroid carcinoma subtypes over time from primarily follicular (1957–1989) to papillary (1990–2004) correlated with the salt iodization program in Nigeria initiated in the early 1990s (**Table 1**). Malignancy rates in goiters in

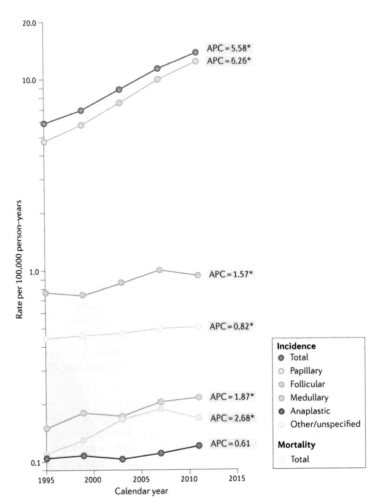

Fig. 4. Thyroid cancer incidence in the United States (1993–2012) according to histology and overall, and overall thyroid cancer mortality incidence. APC, annual percent change. *APC is significantly different from zero (P<.05). (*From* Kitahara CM, Sosa JA. The changing incidence of thyroid cancer. Nat Rev Endocrinol 2016;12:648; with permission.)

iodine-deficient regions however continue to remain high, potentially because of the fact that patients with malignant goiters are more likely to seek medical care than those with nonmalignant goiters.[41] Consequently, Watters and Wall[41] suggest that increased malignancy rates in goiter endemic areas may reflect a lack of access to adequate health services. In addition to this lack of access, the inherent delay in seeking medical care, for both thyroid goiter and carcinoma, has been suggested to play a major role in the high prevalence of malignancy in goiter-endemic regions, with elevated rates of advanced stage disease or anaplastic carcinomas.[42] Bhargav and colleagues[43] further demonstrated this by comparing mean tumor diameters reported by studies from the developing world to those reported from the developed world (3.5 cm vs 1.5 cm, respectively), primarily attributing this difference to delayed patient presentation.

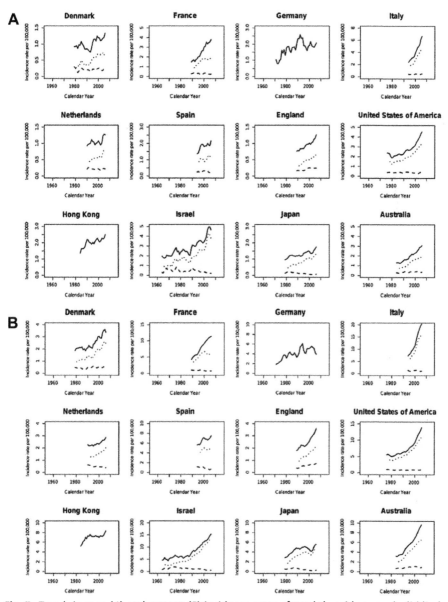

Fig. 5. Trends in men (*A*) and women (*B*) incidence rates of total thyroid cancer (*solid line*), papillary (*dotted line*), and follicular carcinoma (*dashes*). (*From* La Vecchia C, Malvezzi M, Bosetti C, et al. Thyroid cancer mortality and incidence: a global overview. Int J Cancer 2015;136:2193–4; with permission.)

THYROID SURGERY IN THE DEVELOPING WORLD

Guidelines published by the American Thyroid Association[44] aid physicians treating thyroid disease to choose the best evidenced-based option according to the presentation and pathologic condition at hand. However, in low- and middle-income countries, when selecting a treatment option, one must take several factors into

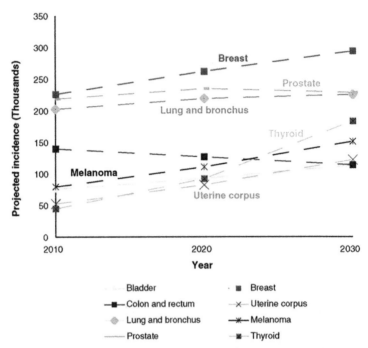

Fig. 6. Projected cancer incidence of the top 8 cancers for both sexes in the United States. (*From* Rahib L, Smith BD, Aizenberg R, et al. Projecting cancer incidence and deaths to 2030: the unexpected burden of thyroid, liver, and pancreas cancers in the United States. Cancer Res 2014;74:2917; with permission.)

consideration that are often taken for granted in high-income countries, such as thyroxine supplies and the cost of a daily thyroxine tablet; increased postoperative complications, morbidity, and mortality due to nonstandardized postoperative management; and inconsistent ability for follow-up appointments, among others.[45,46] Although access to ultrasounds has improved in the developing world, fine-needle aspiration biopsies are rarely performed because of the lack of resources for the performance and analysis, making it that much more difficult to appropriately choose between surgery or observing an enlarged or suspicious nodule.[46] In the eventuality that

Table 1				
Histologic subtypes (papillary and follicular) over time in Ibadan, Nigeria				
Period of Study	**Papillary (%)**	**Follicular (%)**	**Total Thyroid Carcinoma**	**P Value**
1990–2004	35.7	24.8	157	—
1980–1989	27.3	35.8	165	.05
1965–1984[a]	45.4	44.5	137	Not significant
1957–1970[b]	18	60	125	<.00005

[a] Thomas JO, Ogunbiyi JO. Thyroid cancers in Ibadan, Nigeria. East Afr Med J 1995;72:231–3.
[b] Olurin EO, Itayemi S, Oluwasanmi J, et al. The pattern of thyroid gland disease in Ibadan. Niger Med J 1973;3:58–65.
From Woodruff SL, Arowolo OA, Akute OO, et al. Global variation in the pattern of differentiated thyroid cancer. Am J Surg 2010;200:464; with permission.

a thyroid lobectomy or subtotal thyroidectomy is performed, if disease recurs or thyroid cancer is incidentally identified, further surgery may pose a significant challenge, especially if the surgeon is not accustomed to more advanced and complex revision thyroid surgery. It is clear that, especially in the developing world, there is need for individualized care by experienced surgeons to properly manage surgical thyroid disease, taking into account the resources of the patient and the local medical environment.

SOCIOECONOMIC BURDEN OF DISEASE

Rising thyroid disease incidence rates, more specifically that of thyroid cancer, will bring forth a mounting societal and economic impact worldwide. In the United States alone, the increase in cost for thyroid disease management is estimated to triple by 2030 and reach the 3.5 billion dollar mark annually.[23] Furthermore, Ramsey and colleagues[47] examined the rate of bankruptcy in a large cancer population, reporting that patients with thyroid cancer had the highest incidence of bankruptcy and were 3.5 times at higher risk of filing for bankruptcy than for persons without cancer. The latter finding may be associated with the fact that patients with thyroid cancer are often of young age and are more likely to have a high debt-to-income ratio, while being less likely to have access to high-quality health insurance, and not qualifying for Medicare and social security benefits.[48]

A recent international survey[49] on perioperative practices in thyroid surgery evaluated, among other issues, the use of various tools by surgeons that can significantly increase the cost associated with thyroid surgery. For example, although the use of nonconventional and often significantly more expensive approaches such as robotic-assisted thyroid surgery or distant access approaches has been reported in several centers around the world, their prevalence in the global thyroid surgery stage is minimal and will likely remain as such.[49] Even novel hemostatic devices, such as the harmonic scalpel or the electrothermal bipolar vessel sealing system, are used by a minority of thyroid surgeons, partly because of their elevated cost. With increasing diagnosis of thyroid cancer and increasing use of technology in thyroid surgery across the developed world, it may be assumed that the economic burden of thyroid disease will continue to escalate. Ambulatory/outpatient thyroid surgery for appropriate patients in high-resource settings has been proposed as a strategy that may decrease the overall economic cost of thyroid surgery without negatively affecting outcomes.[50,51] This practice is primarily seen in private institutions in the United States,[49] although additional health care institutions and countries may follow suit with further supporting data.

The developing world continues to demonstrate a growing economic disparity,[52] and as previously stated, the burden of thyroid disease is often the greatest in these regions of the world.[53] For thyroid cancer, necessary resources for adequate patient care include surgical facilities with properly trained thyroid surgeons, endocrinologists, access to biochemical laboratories, and access to basic medications, such as thyroxine, calcium, and vitamin D. In addition, the expertise of ancillary medical professionals is often necessary. For example, skilled speech pathologists may help patients dealing with postoperative vocal cord paralysis. In the vast majority of Sub-Saharan African countries, the rate of such professionals are in the range of 0 to 0.6 per 100,000 people,[54] and unfortunately, these rates remain unchanged, if not even decreased over the last few years.[55] Training new medical and paramedical staff is of utmost importance in developing countries, in addition to significant effort toward enticing these trained professionals to remain in low-resource environments. This retention will guarantee a high degree of clinical and surgical intuition coupled with an understanding of the local humanitarian and socioeconomic factors involved in the care of thyroid disease and its long-term consequences in developing countries.[56] By improving access to care for patients with thyroid disease through the development of infrastructure, iodination programs, and standardized resource-appropriate patient management, significant costs savings can be achieved in terms of societal quality of life and a healthier workforce.

REFERENCES

1. Garber JR, Cobin RH, Gharib H, et al. Clinical practice guidelines for hypothyroidism in adults: cosponsored by the American Association of Clinical Endocrinologists and the American Thyroid Association. Endocr Pract 2012;18: 988–1028.
2. American Cancer Society. Cancer Facts & Figures 2016 [Annual report].
3. Ferlay J, Soerjomataram I, Ervik M, et al. GLOBOCAN 2012 v1.0, cancer incidence and mortality worldwide: IARC CancerBase No. 11. Available at: http://globocan.iarc.fr/Pages/summary_table_pop_prev_sel.aspx. Accessed June 20, 2017.
4. Zimmermann MB. Iodine deficiency. Endocr Rev 2009;30:376–408.
5. Zimmermann MB, Andersson M. Update on iodine status worldwide. Curr Opin Endocrinol Diabetes Obes 2012;19:382–7.
6. Gastner MT, Newman M. Iodine deficiency deaths. Available at: http://www.worldmapper.org/display_extra.php?selected=415. Accessed June 20, 2017.
7. Feldt-Rasmussen U. Iodine and cancer. Thyroid 2001;11:483–6.
8. Walker SP, Wachs TD, Gardner JM, et al. Child development: risk factors for adverse outcomes in developing countries. Lancet 2007;369:145–57.
9. Aburto N, Abudou M, Candeias V, et al. Effect and safety of salt iodization to prevent iodine deficiency disorders: a systematic review with meta-analyses. WHO eLibrary of Evidence for Nutrition Actions (eLENA) 2014.
10. Zimmermann MB, Galetti V. Iodine intake as a risk factor for thyroid cancer: a comprehensive review of animal and human studies. Thyroid Res 2015;8:8.
11. Miccoli P, Minuto MN, Galleri D, et al. Incidental thyroid carcinoma in a large series of consecutive patients operated on for benign thyroid disease. ANZ J Surg 2006;76:123–6.
12. Smith JJ, Chen X, Schneider DF, et al. Cancer after thyroidectomy: a multi-institutional experience with 1,523 patients. J Am Coll Surg 2013;216:571–7 [discussion: 577–9].
13. Lasithiotakis K, Grisbolaki E, Koutsomanolis D, et al. Indications for surgery and significance of unrecognized cancer in endemic multinodular goiter. World J Surg 2012;36:1286–92.
14. Nmadu PT, Mabogunje OA. The risk of cancer in endemic multinodular goitre. Cent Afr J Med 1991;37:242–4.
15. Rumstadt B, Klein B, Kirr H, et al. Thyroid surgery in Burkina Faso, West Africa: experience from a surgical help program. World J Surg 2008;32:2627–30.
16. Luo J, McManus C, Chen H, et al. Are there predictors of malignancy in patients with multinodular goiter? J Surg Res 2012;174:207–10.
17. Rios A, Rodriguez JM, Galindo PJ, et al. Surgical treatment of multinodular goiter in young patients. Endocrine 2005;27:245–52.

18. Dralle H, Lorenz K, Machens A. State of the art: surgery for endemic goiter–a plea for individualizing the extent of resection instead of heading for routine total thyroidectomy. Langenbecks Arch Surg 2011;396:1137–43.
19. Stoll SJ, Pitt SC, Liu J, et al. Thyroid hormone replacement after thyroid lobectomy. Surgery 2009;146:554–8 [discussion: 558–60].
20. Vaiman M, Nagibin A, Hagag P, et al. Hypothyroidism following partial thyroidectomy. Otolaryngol Head Neck Surg 2008;138:98–100.
21. Agarwal G, Aggarwal V. Is total thyroidectomy the surgical procedure of choice for benign multinodular goiter? An evidence-based review. World J Surg 2008; 32:1313–24.
22. Donohoe O, Kintu-Luwaga R, Bolger J, et al. A prospective analysis of thyroidectomy outcomes in a resource-limited setting. World J Surg 2015;39:1708–11.
23. Lubitz CC, Kong CY, McMahon PM, et al. Annual financial impact of well-differentiated thyroid cancer care in the United States. Cancer 2014;120: 1345–52.
24. Chen AY, Jemal A, Ward EM. Increasing incidence of differentiated thyroid cancer in the United States, 1988-2005. Cancer 2009;115:3801–7.
25. Kilfoy BA, Zheng T, Holford TR, et al. International patterns and trends in thyroid cancer incidence, 1973-2002. Cancer Causes Control 2009;20:525–31.
26. La Vecchia C, Malvezzi M, Bosetti C, et al. Thyroid cancer mortality and incidence: a global overview. Int J Cancer 2015;136:2187–95.
27. Magrath I, Epelman S. Cancer in adolescents and young adults in countries with limited resources. Curr Oncol Rep 2013;15:332–46.
28. Morris LG, Sikora AG, Tosteson TD, et al. The increasing incidence of thyroid cancer: the influence of access to care. Thyroid 2013;23:885–91.
29. Davies L, Welch HG. Increasing incidence of thyroid cancer in the United States, 1973-2002. JAMA 2006;295:2164–7.
30. Kitahara CM, Sosa JA. The changing incidence of thyroid cancer. Nat Rev Endocrinol 2016;12:646–53.
31. Rahib L, Smith BD, Aizenberg R, et al. Projecting cancer incidence and deaths to 2030: the unexpected burden of thyroid, liver, and pancreas cancers in the United States. Cancer Res 2014;74:2913–21.
32. Ahn HS, Kim HJ, Welch HG. Korea's thyroid-cancer "epidemic"–screening and overdiagnosis. N Engl J Med 2014;371:1765–7.
33. Ahn HS, Welch HG. South Korea's thyroid-cancer "epidemic"–turning the tide. N Engl J Med 2015;373:2389–90.
34. Lim H, Devesa SS, Sosa JA, et al. Trends in thyroid cancer incidence and mortality in the United States, 1974-2013. JAMA 2017;317:1338–48.
35. Kitahara CM, Devesa SS, Sosa JA. Increases in thyroid cancer incidence and mortality-reply. JAMA 2017;318:390–1.
36. Mazonakis M, Tzedakis A, Damilakis J, et al. Thyroid dose from common head and neck CT examinations in children: is there an excess risk for thyroid cancer induction? Eur Radiol 2007;17:1352–7.
37. Bounacer A, Wicker R, Caillou B, et al. High prevalence of activating ret proto-oncogene rearrangements, in thyroid tumors from patients who had received external radiation. Oncogene 1997;15:1263–73.
38. Araque DVP, Bleyer A, Brito JP. Thyroid cancer in adolescents and young adults. Future Oncol 2017;13(14):1253–61.
39. Davies L, Morris LG, Haymart M, et al. American Association of Clinical Endocrinologists and American College of Endocrinology disease state clinical review: the increasing incidence of thyroid cancer. Endocr Pract 2015;21:686–96.

40. Woodruff SL, Arowolo OA, Akute OO, et al. Global variation in the pattern of differentiated thyroid cancer. Am J Surg 2010;200:462–6.
41. Watters DA, Wall J. Thyroid surgery in the tropics. ANZ J Surg 2007;77:933–40.
42. Bakiri F, Djemli FK, Mokrane LA, et al. The relative roles of endemic goiter and socioeconomic development status in the prognosis of thyroid carcinoma. Cancer 1998;82:1146–53.
43. Bhargav PR, Mishra A, Agarwal G, et al. Long-term outcome of differentiated thyroid carcinoma: experience in a developing country. World J Surg 2010;34:40–7.
44. Haugen BR, Alexander EK, Bible KC, et al. 2015 American Thyroid Association Management guidelines for adult patients with thyroid nodules and differentiated thyroid cancer: the American Thyroid Association Guidelines Task Force on thyroid nodules and differentiated thyroid cancer. Thyroid 2016;26:1–133.
45. Gaitan E, Nelson NC, Poole GV. Endemic goiter and endemic thyroid disorders. World J Surg 1991;15:205–15.
46. Burali G, Martin OD, Fiorini FR, et al. Total thyroidectomy in North Uganda: a cultural and socio-economic challenge for an African Country. J Thyroid Disord Ther 2016;5:206.
47. Ramsey S, Blough D, Kirchhoff A, et al. Washington State cancer patients found to be at greater risk for bankruptcy than people without a cancer diagnosis. Health Aff (Millwood) 2013;32:1143–52.
48. Sturgeon C. Patients with thyroid cancer are at higher risk of bankruptcy than patients with other types of cancer, or those without cancer. Clin Thyroidol 2013;25:150–1.
49. Maniakas A, Christopoulos A, Bissada E, et al. Perioperative practices in thyroid surgery: an international survey. Head Neck 2017;39:1296–305.
50. Meltzer C, Klau M, Gurushanthaiah D, et al. Safety of outpatient thyroid and parathyroid surgery: a propensity score-matched study. Otolaryngol Head Neck Surg 2016;154(5):789–96.
51. Grubey JS, Raji Y, Duke WS, et al. Outpatient thyroidectomy is safe in the elderly and super-elderly. Laryngoscope 2018;128(1):290–4.
52. Vieira S. Inequality on the rise? United Nations. Available at: http://www.un.org/en/development/desa/policy/wess/wess_bg_papers/bp_wess2013_svieira1.pdf. Accessed July 22, 2017.
53. Jafari A, Campbell D, Campbell BH, et al. Thyroid surgery in a resource-limited setting. Otolaryngol Head Neck Surg 2017;156:464–71.
54. Fagan JJ, Jacobs M. Survey of ENT services in Africa: need for a comprehensive intervention. Glob Health Action 2009.
55. Mulwafu W, Ensink R, Kuper H, et al. Survey of ENT services in sub-Saharan Africa: little progress between 2009 and 2015. Glob Health Action 2017;10:1289736.
56. Baxi M, Shetty KJ, Baxi J, et al. Need for an individualized and aggressive management of multinodular goiters of endemic zones by specially trained surgeons: experience in western Nepal. World J Surg 2006;30:2101–9 [discussion: 2110–1].

Workforce Considerations, Training, and Diseases in Africa

Johannes J. Fagan, MBChB, M.Med., FCS (ORL)

KEYWORDS

• Sub-Saharan Africa • Otolaryngology • Training • Fellowships • Workforce

KEY POINTS

- Sub-Saharan Africa (SSA) has extreme shortages of otolaryngologists, speech pathologists, and audiologists; a lack of training opportunities; and a paucity of otolaryngology services.
- In addition to diseases commonly encountered in Western countries, patients have otolaryngology pathologic complications related to the human immunodeficiency virus, tuberculosis, malaria, and trauma.
- Less than 5% of the population has access to timely, safe, affordable surgery.
- It is critical that training centers of excellence be established in SSA.

INTRODUCTION

Sub-Saharan Africa (SSA) has extreme shortages of otolaryngologists, speech pathologists and audiologists, a lack of training opportunities, and a paucity of otolaryngology services (**Table 1**).[1,2] The population of SSA was 800 million in 2007; the United Nations predicts a population of 1.5 to 2 billion by 2050.[3] The inadequacy of services will be aggravated by this rapid population growth. Otolaryngology services in SSA also face an increasing burden of diseases associated with aging because the number of older people has doubled since 1990 and is projected to more than triple between 2015 and 2050[4] (see **Table 1**).

DISEASES

In addition to diseases commonly encountered in Western countries, patients in SSA present with otolaryngology complications related to, among others, the human immunodeficiency virus (HIV), tuberculosis (TB), malaria, and trauma. Patients are

---

Disclosure: The author has nothing to disclose.
Division of Otorhinolaryngology, Faculty of Health Sciences, University of Cape Town, H53 OMB Groote Schuur Hospital, Observatory, Cape Town 7925, South Africa
E-mail address: johannes.fagan@uct.ac.za

Otolaryngol Clin N Am 51 (2018) 643–649
https://doi.org/10.1016/j.otc.2018.01.009
oto.theclinics.com

Table 1
Number of ear, nose, and throat surgeons, new graduates per annum and training opportunities in 2015

Country	Number of Ear, Nose, and Throat (ENT) Surgeons	ENT Training Centers	New ENTs per Year	Audiology Training Centers	Speech Training Centers
Burundi	6	1	1	—	—
Cameroon	35	1	5	—	—
Democratic Republic of Congo	18	1	2	—	—
Ethiopia	22	1	4	—	—
Ghana	27	2	2	Yes	—
Guinea Conakry	6	3	5	—	—
Kenya	76	1	1	Yes	Yes
Lesotho	2	—	—	—	—
Madagascar	15	1	1	—	—
Malawi	2	1	0	—	—
Mali	15	1	4	—	—
Nigeria	140	37	5	—	—
Rwanda	8	1	2	—	—
South Africa	246	9	6	Yes	Yes
Senegal	15	1	4	—	—
Sudan	105	0	10	—	—
Swaziland	3	—	—	—	—
Tanzania	18	2	3	—	—
Togo	8	1	Unknown	—	Yes
Uganda	35	2	4	—	—
Zambia	7	—	—	—	—
Zimbabwe	8	1	2	—	—

Data from Mulwafu W, Ensink R, Kuper H, et al. Survey of ENT services in Sub-Saharan Africa: little progress between 2009 and 2015. Glob Health Action 2017. https://doi.org/10.1080/16549716.2017.1289736.

more likely to present with advanced cancers (many of which are incurable), complicated cholesteatoma, and infections of the middle ear and sinuses.

Human Immunodeficiency Virus

SSA harbors greater than 70% of the global burden of HIV.[5] Up to 80% of HIV-positive patients will develop otolaryngology manifestations of HIV (**Table 2**).[6]

Tuberculosis

SSA has the highest TB burden globally, and greater than 50% of TB patients are coinfected with HIV. TB may affect the upper and lower aerodigestive tracts; or present with lymphadenitis, cold abscesses, and scrofula; meningitis, causing sensorineural hearing loss (SNHL); and TB of the middle ear, mastoid, and temporal bone, sometimes causing facial nerve paralysis or mastoiditis. Patients with multidrug-resistant TB require ototoxic drugs, the levels of which are not monitored in resource-limited settings, hence causing SNHL. The risk of ototoxicity is increased in HIV-positive TB patients.[7]

Table 2	
Some common otolaryngology manifestations of the human immunodeficiency virus	
Infections	TB
	Candidiasis
	Herpes simplex
	Herpes zoster
	Invasive fungal sinusitis
Lymphoreticular	Persistent generalized lymphadenopathy
	Adenotonsillar hypertrophy
Neoplasms	Non-Hodgkin lymphoma
	Kaposi sarcoma
	Conjunctival squamous cell carcinoma
Oral	Hairy leukoplakia
	Ulcers: aphthous, herpes
	Gingivitis, periodontitis, angular cheilitis
Otological	Chronic serous otitis media
	Sensorineural hearing loss
Neurologic	Cranial nerve palsies
Salivary	Xerostomia
	Benign lymphoepithelial lesion
	Lymphoepithelial cysts

Data from Iacovou E, Vlastarakos PV, Papacharalampous G, et al. Diagnosis and treatment of HIV-associated manifestations in otolaryngology. Infect Dis Rep 2012;4(1):e9.

Malaria

Malaria is endemic in much of SSA. Both malaria and quinine can cause SNHL.

Pediatric Hearing Loss

More than 1.2 million children in SSA ages 5 to 14 years have bilateral moderate to severe hearing loss.[8] Prevalence rates of pediatric hearing loss range from 2.2% to 9.2%.[8] Limited access to antenatal, perinatal, and postnatal care increases the risk of congenital hearing loss. Other causes of SNHL include measles, meningitis, viral infections, and ototoxic drugs.[8] It has been estimated that proper management of measles, mumps, meningitis, rubella, and otitis media could halve the number of hearing loss cases in developing countries[8]; however, vaccination programs are nonexistent in many regions.

Aging Population

Noncommunicable diseases associated with aging include cancers of the head and neck, and SNHL.

Noise Exposure

Due to a lack of industrial regulations for hearing protection, many workers are exposed to high levels of noise, causing SNHL.

Head and Neck Cancer

It is predicted that by 2030, 70% of cancers will be in the developing world.[9] This increase has been attributed to an aging population, population growth, and reduction in deaths from communicable diseases. In Africa, there were approximately 681,000 new cancer cases and 512,000 deaths in 2008; this is predicted to increase to 1.27 million cases and 0.97 million deaths as a consequence of population growth and aging.[10]

Trauma

Blunt and penetrating head injuries cause a range of otolaryngology pathologic complications. The World Health Organization (WHO) estimates that almost 90% of deaths due to injury occur in low-income and middle-income countries.[11] SSA has a head injury incidence of 150 to 170 per 100,000 population due to motor vehicle accidents compared with the global rate of 106 per 100,000.[12] Most accidents occur in rural areas that are poorly equipped to deal with trauma victims.

WORKFORCE CONSIDERATIONS

Prevention and management of otolaryngology diseases requires primary health care (including obstetric and perinatal care, and immunizations) delivered by nurses, clinical officers, and general medical practitioners, as well as specialized care by otolaryngologists, audiologists, speech pathologists, oncologists, and related specialties. The absence of radiotherapy facilities in 29 out of 52 countries in Africa results in reliance on surgery to treat cancers of the head and neck in most SSA countries.[13] Yet less than 5% of the population in SSA has access to timely, safe, affordable surgery.[14]

Audits of workforce availability in SSA in 2009 and 2015 report a severe shortage of otolaryngologists, audiologists, and speech pathologists, as well as limited or no access to even basic surgical procedures and equipment in most of the countries polled, with a concentration of services in urban areas.[1,2] Malawi has only 2 otolaryngologists for 18 million people and has, therefore, instituted a training program for ear, nose, and throat (ENT) clinical officers to provide basic diagnostic and surgical care in underserved areas.[2]

It is essential that SSA invest in education and training of nurses, clinical officers, and general medical practitioners, as well as otolaryngologists, audiologists, speech pathologists, oncologists, and allied specialists such as anesthetists.

TRAINING

Surgeons in SSA face different challenges than those in developed countries. They apply different selection criteria due to overwhelming burdens of disease, unreliable follow-up, and limited radiotherapy. They frequently lack modern surgical technology, frozen section procedures, blood products, operating time, good anesthesia, and intensive care support. They adapt modern surgical principles and techniques to a lower-technology practice. The ideal training model would provide appropriate training that is affordable to trainees and that leads to the establishment of otolaryngology centers of excellence that can teach and train otolaryngologists, audiologists, and speech pathologists. Such training can be achieved in several ways, some of which are complimentary (see later discussion).

Training in Developed Countries

Although developed countries provide excellent training, their training is becoming less appropriate for SSA as the gap in technology and resources widens. Therefore, providing training in SSA is appropriate in terms of pathologic assessment, management algorithms, technology, and surgical techniques. Trainees who train in SSA are also likely to remain in SSA as opposed to those who train in developed countries; 86% (16 out of 18) of ENT surgeons from SSA (other than South Africa) who trained at the University of Cape Town have remained in SSA, as have all 12 University of Cape Town head and neck surgical fellows.

Otolaryngology Training in Sub-Saharan Africa

Training presents significant challenges in many countries in SSA: inadequate operating time, many trainees are self-funded, lack of exposure to more complex surgery,[1,2] poor access to temporal bone laboratories, and lack of allied services such as audiology, speech pathology, and oncology.[1,2]

Another challenge is how to establish new training programs when countries lack a critical mass of ENT surgeons to run a program. New programs in Rwanda and Zimbabwe used different start-up models. The Rwandan program was initiated in 2010 with the support of German otolaryngologists.[15] German ENT doctors lecture, do surgery, and provide training in the outpatient clinic. Rwanda bears the costs of board and lodging. Flights, medical equipment, and materials are financed by charity. Examinations are conducted in Kigali, with external examiners from South Africa and elsewhere to ensure standard setting. The first 2 ENT specialists graduated in 2014. Unlike the Rwandan program, the first trainees of the new Zimbabwean training program underwent 3 months' surgical intensive care training in Cape Town and ENT training in Harare. They took the examinations of the College of Otolaryngologists of South Africa. The first 2 ENT surgeons qualified in 2016. The South African examination system was, therefore, used while they built their program and examination system.

Another potential training avenue is the College of Surgeons of East, Central, and Southern Africa (COSECSA). COSECSA is an independent body that advances postgraduate surgical training in Burundi, Ethiopia, Kenya, Malawi, Mozambique, Rwanda, Tanzania, Uganda, Zambia, and Zimbabwe. It provides a common surgical training program in accredited hospitals and a single set of examinations. It is ideally suited to countries lacking a critical mass of teachers and examiners. Although well-established for disciplines such as orthopedics, general surgery, and obstetrics and gynecology, otolaryngology has not yet graduated specialists through COSECSA.

Subspecialty Training in Sub-Saharan Africa

Subspecialty training is important if levels of clinical service, teaching, and research are to be increased. There are only 3 fellowship training programs in SSA.

The University of Cape Town Karl Storz Fellowship in Advanced Head and Neck Surgery was established in 2005. Its format is similar to American fellowships. It is a 12-month clinical fellowship and surgical exposure compares favorably with programs in the United States.[16] The first 12 fellows from Uganda, Kenya, Senegal, Ghana (2), Nigeria (2), Rwanda, Malawi, Tanzania, Zimbabwe, and Ethiopia all returned to teaching hospitals in their home countries to teach others. The University of Cape Town Karl Storz Fellowship in Rhinology and Anterior Skull Base Surgery is currently training its third fellow. Fellows have originated from South Africa, Libya, and Namibia.

The Pan-African Academy of Christian Surgeons (PAACS)–Cameroonian Baptist Convention (CBC)–Hopkins Head and Neck Fellowship program at the Mbingo Baptist Hospital in Northwest Cameroon is a novel outreach-training model. The first fellow from Kenya qualified in 2017; the current fellow is from Ethiopia. It is a cooperative project of the Department of Otolaryngology–Head and Neck Surgery at Johns Hopkins Medical Institutions, the CBC, and the PAACS. It is modeled on the American Head and Neck Society's fellowship programs and is a 1-year, hands-on, surgical and academic training experience. Training is provided by volunteer head and neck surgeons from the United States and a resident ENT surgeon.

Training Through Clinical Missions and Academic Support

The lack of otolaryngologists in SSA presents an opportunity for surgeons from developed countries to collaborate in education and training. This may take the form of workshops that incorporate didactic teaching, cadaver dissections, and live surgery, at both an individual level and through interinstitutional collaborations.[17]

Access to Literature

Many trainees and surgeons in SSA cannot afford journals, pay-for-view journal articles, and textbooks. HINARI was set up by the WHO and provides free access to biomedical and health literature for low-income and middle-income countries (http://www.who.int/hinari/en/). Journals and textbooks generally cater for developed world practice; hence the need for free, Internet-based resources that are appropriate to developing world practice. The "*Open Access Atlas of Otolaryngology Head and Neck Operative Surgery*" and the "*Open Access Guide to Audiology and Hearing Aids for Otolaryngologists*" are examples of free educational resources that are appropriate to low-resource settings (http://www.entdev.uct.ac.za/). It is hoped that societies such as the American Head and Neck Society and American Academy of Otolaryngology Head and Neck Surgery will similarly make all their resources freely available.

REFERENCES

1. Fagan JJ, Jacobs M. Survey of ENT services in Africa: need for a comprehensive intervention. Glob Health Action 2009;2. Available at: http://journals.sfu.ca/coaction/index.php/gha/article/view/1932.
2. Mulwafu W, Ensink R, Kuper H, et al. Survey of ENT services in Sub-Saharan Africa: little progress between 2009 and 2015. Glob Health Action 2017. https://doi.org/10.1080/16549716.2017.1289736.
3. "World population prospects - population division - United Nations". 2015. Available at: Esa.un.org. Accessed April 17, 2017.
4. Report on world population ageing 2015. New York: United Nations, Department of Economic and Social Affairs, Population Division; 2015 (ST/ESA/SER.A/390).
5. Kharsany ABM, Karim QA. HIV infection and AIDS in Sub-Saharan Africa: current status, challenges and opportunities. Open AIDS J 2016;10:34–48.
6. Iacovou E, Vlastarakos PV, Papacharalampous G, et al. Diagnosis and treatment of HIV-associated manifestations in otolaryngology. Infect Dis Rep 2012; 4(1):e9.
7. Harris T, Bardien S, Schaaf HS, et al. Aminoglycoside-induced hearing loss in HIV-positive and HIV-negative multidrug-resistant tuberculosis patients. S Afr Med J 2012;102(6):363–6.
8. Tucci DL, Merson MH, Wilson BS. A summary of the literature on global hearing impairment: current status and priorities for action. Otol Neurotol 2010;31(1): 31–41.
9. Farmer P, Frenk J, Knaul FM, et al. Expansion of cancer care and control in countries of low and middle income: a call to action. Lancet 2010;376(9747):1186–93.
10. Sylla BS, Wild CP. A million Africans a year dying from cancer by 2030: what can cancer research and control offer to the continent? Int J Cancer 2012;130: 245–50.
11. Murray CJL, Lopez AD. The global burden of disease: a comprehensive assessment of mortality and disability; from diseases injuries, and risk factors in 1990 and projected to 2020. Cambridge (MA): Harvard University Press.

12. Odero W, Garner P, Zwi A. Road traffic injuries in developing countries: a comprehensive review of epidemiological studies. Trop Med Int Health 1997;2(5):445–60 [Meta-Analysis Research Support, Non-U.S. Gov't].
13. Abdel-Wahab M, Bourque J-M, Pynda Y, et al. Status of radiotherapy resources in Africa: an international atomic energy agency analysis. Lancet Oncol 2013; 14(4):e168–75. Available at: http://www.thelancet.com/journals/lanonc/article/PIIS1470-2045%2812%2970532-6/fulltext#article_upsell.
14. Alkire BC, Raykar NP, Shrime MG, et al. Global access to surgical care. A modelling study. Lancet Glob Health 2015;3:e316–23.
15. Helping people to help themselves–training ENT doctors in Rwanda: interview with Stefan Dazert by Raffaela Römer. 2015. Available at: http://rubin.rub.de/en/featured-topic-conflicts/helping-people-help-themselves-training-ent-doctors-rwanda. Accessed February 16, 2018.
16. Fagan JJ, Zafereo M, Aswani J, et al. Head and neck surgical subspecialty training in Africa. Sustainable models to improve cancer care in developing countries. Head Neck 2016. https://doi.org/10.1002/hed.24591.
17. Fagan JJ, Aswani J, Otiti J, et al. Educational workshops with graduates of the University of Cape Town Karl Storz Head and Neck Surgery Fellowship Program: a model for collaboration in outreach to developing countries. Springerplus 2016; 5(1):1652, eCollection 2016.

Regional Overview of Specific Populations, Workforce Considerations, Training, and Diseases in Latin America

Jose Pablo Stolovitzky, MD[a,b],*, Jacqueline Alvarado, MD[c,d]

KEYWORDS

- Otorhinolaryngology • Latin America • Health care workforce
- Postgraduate training • Manpower shortage

KEY POINTS

- In Latin America, there is a broad range of local health care issues requiring individualized strategies to solve them.
- There are shortages in the otorhinolaryngology workforce in about 50% of the Latin American countries.
- Although all countries in Latin America have at least one residency program, there is a need to increase the number of otorhinolaryngology-trained specialists.
- Health care delivery in public hospitals is deficient because of budgetary constraints and system inefficiencies.
- The cochlear implant programs in Latin America have grown exponentially, particularly in countries where public and private support have been instituted.

REGIONAL OVERVIEW

The Latin American population exceeds 600 million inhabitants and 11 million births per year, with a geographic area well more than 20 million km². The region contains large contrasts ranging from huge industrial compounds to extreme poverty suburbs.[1,2] The gross domestic product ranges from $4884.15 in Nicaragua to $22,316.2 in Chile. Because of these disparities, health care strategies and medical education should be adapted to the characteristics of each nation and location.[2]

Disclosure Statement: The authors have nothing to disclose.
[a] Department of Otolaryngology, Emory University School of Medicine, 201 Dowman Drive, Atlanta, GA 30322, USA; [b] ENT of Georgia North, 5673 Peachtree Dunwoody Road, Suite 150, Atlanta, GA 30342, USA; [c] Pan-American Society of Otorhinolaryngology–Head and Neck Surgery, Atlanta, GA, USA; [d] Venezuelan Society of Otolaryngology, Caracas, Venezuela
* Corresponding author. Department of Otolaryngology, Emory University School of Medicine, Atlanta, GA.
E-mail address: STOL@ENTOFGA.COM

Otolaryngol Clin N Am 51 (2018) 651–658
https://doi.org/10.1016/j.otc.2018.01.015
0030-6665/18/© 2018 Elsevier Inc. All rights reserved.

oto.theclinics.com

Otorhinolaryngology is a growing specialty in Latin America, with a need for training and improved public health care as well as enhanced data collection and reporting. According to the World Bank's 2011 data, a high percentage of Latin Americans live in rural areas and most otorhinolaryngologists are concentrated in the major cities.[3]

Recently, in order to clarify this situation, an independent survey was conducted both online and in person among 25 Latin American otorhinolaryngology (ORL) leaders from 18 Latin American countries that revealed some interesting data that shed light on the specific needs, similarities, and differences of each nation in the region (Alvarado J, Stolovitzky P. State of Otorhinolaryngology in Latin America: a leaders' survey, unpublished data, 2017).

DISEASES
Upper Respiratory Tract Infections

Similar to most regions around the world, upper respiratory tract infections are quite frequent in Latin America[4]; 80% of children in the region have had at least one episode of acute otitis media before 5 years of age, and 80% of these are due to pneumococcus or *Haemophilus influenzae* type b.[5] Venezuela and Peru are the countries of the region with the highest prevalence of rhinosinusitis; most cases are managed by general practitioners, and only 29% are treated by otorhinolaryngologists.[4]

The rate of pediatric rhinosinusitis in Brazil ranges from 5% to 15% per year. The rate of complications is estimated at around 1% to 5% throughout Latin America. Mortality due to this disease is less than 1% in all of these countries (Alvarado J, Stolovitzky P. State of Otorhinolaryngology in Latin America: a leaders' survey, unpublished data, 2017).

Chronic Suppurative Otitis Media

The estimated global incidence rate of chronic suppurative otitis media is 4.76 per one thousand people for a total of 31 million cases, with 22.6% of these cases occurring annually in children less than 5 years of age. The Andean region in Latin America is the area with the lowest incidence (1.70 per 1000), followed by high-income Asia Pacific (3.02) and high-income North America (3.06).[6]

There are limited data from the region on the prevalence of otitis media–associated hearing impairment, which has a global prevalence (defined as permanent 25 dB hearing loss for the best ear) of 30.82 per 10,000 inhabitants. One study from Latin America exhibits a low prevalence ranging from 4.95 to 5.30 per 10,000.[6] The Global Burden of Disease project estimates the rate of otitis media (all cases) to range from 11.39 per 10,000 in the tropical regions of Latin America to 14.22 per 10,000 in the Andes.[7]

Pediatric Hearing Loss

Hearing loss is a multifactorial condition that impairs the quality of life.[8] According to the United Nations Children's Fund, the world hearing loss prevalence in children is 2.6 per 1000.[1] The number of cases in Latin America and the Caribbean is estimated between 1 and 5 per 1000 live births[9]; however, few of them are identified early because of the poor implementation of adequate and efficient hearing screening.[1] Argentina, Brazil, Colombia, and Cuba have hearing impairment records and use nonstructured but focalized newborn hearing screening protocols. Chile has laws and early hearing loss detection programs, whereas Costa Rica relies on the Association for the Detection and Intervention of Deafness.[9] The percentage of hearing loss in Brazil is 5.1% and 13.0% in Nicaragua, whereas the number of people with a hearing impairment in Panama is 20,500 (Alvarado J, Stolovitzky P. State of Otorhinolaryngology in Latin America: a leaders' survey, unpublished data, 2017).

A study reported that 32% of autistic children in Latin American countries have one easily treatable cause of hearing loss, suggesting the need to establish rational diagnostic and follow-up programs.[10]

Nicaragua analyzed the cost and the implications of implementing newborn hearing screening in the rural areas and concluded that the detection of otoacoustic emissions is both feasible and cost-effective. Guatemala, a country similar to Nicaragua in terms of its economy and geography, implemented an infant grant screening system using otoacoustic emissions in 2004.[11]

Cochlear Implant

Cochlear implant programs started in Latin America around 1985.[12] The development of cochlear implant programs in Latin America has moved forward exponentially. By 2005, the total number of patients with implants was 3773.[13] It is estimated that the number of cochlear implants exceeded 25,000 in 2017 (Alvarado J, Stolovitzky P. State of Otorhinolaryngology in Latin America: a leaders' survey, unpublished data). The countries with the greatest number of implants are Argentina, Brazil, Colombia, Mexico, and Venezuela.[14] In Colombia, Argentina, Brazil, and Cuba, implant programs are government financed, whereas in Mexico, Peru, Venezuela, Chile, and Uruguay, designated stated funds are added to private funding.[14]

In spite of these initiatives, it has been estimated that the number of children who are deaf who are born in Latin America is 20,000 per year; only 3000 cochlear implants are placed annually, resulting in a significant deficit in terms of treatment.[15]

Head and Neck Cancer

The incidence of oral and oropharyngeal cancer in South America varies, with the highest rates found in Brazil among men. The mortality data in selected South American countries ranges from 0.72 to 6.04 per 100,000.[16] There is remarkable variability in the global incidence of these malignancies, which is attributed to differences in cultural lifestyles that involve tobacco and alcohol use, the two most widely known risk factors for oral cavity cancer, and to the prevalence of human papillomavirus (HPV) infection, which represents the main etiologic risk factor for oropharyngeal cancer.[17,18] The odds ratio (OR) for cigarette smoking (ever-smokers vs never-smokers) was higher in South America (OR, 4.54; 95% confidence interval [CI], 3.89–5.31) than in North America (OR, 2.09; 95% CI, 1.89–2.32).[19]

Data on the prevalence of HPV in the Central and South American region are sparse, and only a few small studies are available (sample sizes ranging from 5 to <250 cases) in which different HPV detection techniques were used. In Argentina, Brazil, and Cuba, the prevalence of HPV ranged from 0% to 19% in oropharyngeal cancer, from 0% to 78% in oral cavity cancer (including Mexico and Venezuela), and from 0.8% to 48.5% in hypopharyngeal and laryngeal cancer (including Chile).[20]

In addition to these risk factors, some South Americans are exposed to mate. The dried leaves and stem lets of the perennial tree *Ilex paraguariensis* (yerba mate) are brewed and consumed as a beverage in many countries in South America, mainly in Argentina, southern Brazil, Paraguay, and Uruguay. Hot mate has been classified as potentially carcinogenic to humans, based on evidence of its apparent association with head and neck squamous cell carcinoma. Claims have been made about the association between repeated thermal injury in the mouth, pharynx, and larynx due to the consumption of very hot mate and cancer; furthermore, some of the chemical components of mate may be carcinogens.[21,22]

Human Immunodeficiency Virus and Tuberculosis

In Latin America, the overall rate of new human immunodeficiency virus (HIV) infections has remained stable between 2010 and 2015. Among adults, a 3% increase in rates of new HIV infections between 2010 and 2015 contrasted sharply with a 20% decline during the previous decade.[23] In 2015, there were an estimated 2 million people living with HIV in this region, an infection prevalence of 0.5%. In the same year, there were an estimated 100,000 new HIV infections and 50,000 deaths from AIDS-related illnesses. In Latin America, around 44,300 children younger than 15 years have HIV.[24]

Access to antiretroviral treatment (ART) across Latin America and the Caribbean is disparate. Treatment coverage was 56% among all people living with HIV in Latin America in 2015 compared with 34% in 2011. Latin America has the highest total expenditure on ART among low- and middle-income countries, with Argentina, Brazil, Chile, Cuba, Guyana, and Mexico providing universal access to HIV treatment. However, treatment coverage varies greatly by country. For example, more than half of all people living with HIV were accessing ART in Argentina (64%), Chile (87%), Costa Rica (56%), and Mexico (59%). By contrast, treatment coverage is just 29% in Bolivia.[25]

AIDS-related deaths in Venezuela have nearly doubled in just 5 years, with a public health crisis severely affecting the government's ability to control the epidemic. The Venezuelan Society of Infectious Diseases stated that supplies of key drugs used for the treatment of HIV are dangerously low and in danger of stock-out.[25]

Retrospective studies suggest that the prevalence of head and neck symptoms in patients with HIV is about 80%. Oral manifestations are the most frequent, followed by neck, sinus, and otological findings.[26] Candidiasis is the most common disease in the mouth of patients with HIV/AIDS. Its estimated prevalence in Latin America is about 40% of oral lesions.[27]

Tuberculosis continues to be a public health threat in Latin America, with an incidence rate of 39.6 per 100,000 inhabitants in the region. HIV, *Mycobacterium tuberculosis* resistant to antituberculosis medications, growing inequalities resulting from increased poverty, and poor health care systems in many countries have all exacerbated the problem of tuberculosis.[27]

ACCESS TO PUBLIC HOSPITALS

Waiting times for surgery in public hospitals are associated with the efficiency of health care systems. Long waiting times in Latin American hospitals not only reflect a deficient service but also an increased risk of potential complications, with the subsequent decline in quality of life and increased costs for the health care system (Alvarado J, Stolovitzky P. State of Otorhinolaryngology in Latin America: a leaders' survey, unpublished data, 2017).

The authors' survey demonstrated that the waiting times observed for elective surgery in public hospitals exhibit a wide variability from country to country (Alvarado J, Stolovitzky P. State of Otorhinolaryngology in Latin America: a leaders' survey, unpublished data, 2017) (**Table 1**).

OTORHINOLARYNGOLOGY HEALTH CARE WORKFORCE

There is ample evidence about the imbalances in terms of shortages, composition, and distribution of health care resources in Latin America. The workforce of otorhinolaryngologists (ORL) was evaluated as well as the number of graduate specialization programs in some Latin American countries.

Table 1
Waiting times observed for elective surgery in public hospitals

Country	Waiting Times for Surgery (wk)
Argentina	2–8
Brazil	12–24
Colombia	8
Costa Rica	4
Ecuador	24
Guatemala	16
Honduras	24
Nicaragua	4–12
Panama	12–24
Peru	2–6
Venezuela	4–24

Table 2 shows the rates of ORL doctors per 100,000 inhabitants in different countries of the region (Alvarado J, Stolovitzky P. State of Otorhinolaryngology in Latin America: a leaders' survey, unpublished data, 2017).

The World Health Organization (WHO) recommends 2 otolaryngologist specialists per 100,000 inhabitants (heavy line in **Table 2**), and the results of the survey indicate

Table 2
Rates of otorhinolaryngology doctors in Latin American countries

Country	Population as of August 2017	ORL	ORL Rate per 100,000 Inhabitants
Chile	8,357,784	500	6.0
Argentina	44,379,539	2500	5.6
Mexico	129,678,021	6000	4.6
Uruguay	3,455,803	120	3.5
Brazil	207,848,115	5.703	2.7
Costa Rica	4,924,391	104	2.1
Panama	4,066,879	80	1.9[a]
Peru	32,260,264	600	1.9
Venezuela	32,047,287	600	1.9
Paraguay	6,828,429	100	1.5
Colombia	49,251,603	700	1.4
El Salvador	6,163,786	80	1.3
Ecuador	16,682,331	200	1.2
Nicaragua	6,233,840	72	1.2
Dominican Republic	10,807,990	110	1.0
Bolivia	11,082,513	100	0.9
Honduras	8,329,025	78	0.9
Guatemala	17,066,994	65	0.4

[a] World Health Organization's recommendation.

Adapted from Vásquez-Garcia J, Salas-Hernández S, Padilla Rogelio, et al. Respiratory health in Latin America: number of specialists and human resources training. Arch Bronconeumol 2014;50(1):36; with permission.

that several countries have less than this recommended rate (Alvarado J, Stolovitzky P. State of Otorhinolaryngology in Latin America: a leaders' survey, unpublished data). The findings showed that only Chile, Argentina, Mexico, and Uruguay have higher rates. By comparison, in the United States, the rate was 3.26 ORL doctors per 100,000 inhabitants in 2009.

POSTGRADUATE TRAINING

Although all countries in Latin America have at least one residency program, the data shown earlier indicate there is a need to increase the number of ORL-trained specialists (Alvarado J, Stolovitzky P. State of Otorhinolaryngology in Latin America: a leaders' survey, unpublished data, 2017). According to a study carried out by the WHO in 14 Latin American countries in 2011, ORL is a specialty with 3 to 4 years of residency, depending on the particular country. In Cuba, Paraguay, and Uruguay, the residency program is 3 years, whereas in Colombia, Costa Rica, and Honduras, the residency is 4 years.

Although a few countries in the region offer a comprehensive range of subspecialty training, the increased demand for advanced education requires otorhinolaryngologists to seek training abroad in the form of observerships or fellowships (Alvarado J, Stolovitzky P. State of Otorhinolaryngology in Latin America: a leaders' survey, unpublished data, 2017).

SUMMARY

As a growing specialty in Latin America, otorhinolaryngology has a shortage in most countries in the region. There is a definitive need to increase the number of trained ORL specialists and improve the available resources in tertiary public hospitals.

ACKNOWLEDGMENTS

The authors thank the otorhinolaryngologist leaders for their contributions to the State of Otorhinolaryngology in Latin America Survey: Dra Tania Sih (Brazil), Dr Carlos Boccio (Argentina), Dr Hector De La Garza (Mexico), Dr Domingo Tsuji (Brazil), Dr Enrique Mansilla (Argentina), Dr Juan David Bedolla (Colombia), Dr Miguel Parra (Colombia), Dr Arturo Alanis, (Mexico), Dr Mauricio Buitrago(Costa Rica), Dr Carlos Stott(Chile), Dr Rodrigo Castrillon(Ecuador), Dra Amarilis Melendez (Panama), Dra Carla Carcamo (Honduras), Dra Daliza Gonzalez (Nicaragua), Dra Claudia Vasquez (Perú), Dr Roberto Gutierrez (Bolivia), Dr Carlos Mena(Paraguay), Dra Nydia Amenabar(Guatemala), Dr Rodolfo Lugo (Mexico), Dra Rolanda Gil (Costa Rica), Dr Andres Saibene (Uruguay), Dr Adan Fuentes (El Salvador), Dra Rubidia Escobar (El Salvador), Dra Ligia Acosta (Venezuela), Dr Freddy Ferrera (Dominican Republic).

The authors also thank Ximena Sanchez and Martha Florez de Briceño for their medical writing and editorial support.

REFERENCES

1. Gerner de Garcia B, Gaffney C, Chacon S, et al. Overview of newborn hearing screening activities in Latin America. Rev Panam Salud Publica 2011;29(3): 145–52.
2. Pulido PA, Cravioto A, Pereda A, et al. Changes, trends and challenges of medical education in Latin America. Med Teach 2006;28(1):24–9.
3. Wagner R, Fagan J. Survey of otolaryngology services in Central America: need for a comprehensive intervention. Otolaryngol Head Neck Surg 2013; 149(5):674–8.

4. Neffen H, Mello JF, Sole D, et al. Nasal allergies in the Latin American population: results from the allergies in Latin America survey. Allergy Asthma Proc 2010; 31(3):9–27.

5. Sanchez F, Alvarado J, Acosta L, et al. IV Consenso Venezolano en Infecciones Otorrinolaringológicas. Acta Otorrinolaringológica de Venezuela 2013;(Suppl): 1–117.

6. Monasta L, Ronfani L, Marchetti F, et al. Burden of disease caused by otitis media: systematic review and global estimates. PLoS One 2012;7(4):e36226.

7. Institute of Health Metrics Evaluation - Global burden of disease (GBD-Compare) Website. Available at: https://vizhub.healthdata.org/gbd-compare/. Accessed August 16, 2017.

8. OMS. Sordera y pérdida de audición. Washington, DC: Organization Mundial De La Salud; 2017. Available at: http://www.who.int/mediacentre/factsheets/fs300/es/. Accessed August 16, 2017.

9. Albertz N, Cardemil F, Rahal M, et al. Programa de tamizaje universal e intervención precoz (PTUIP) en hipoacusia sensorioneural bilateral congénita: tarea pendiente desde la perspectiva de políticas públicas de salud en Chile. Rev Med Chil 2013;141(8):1057–63. Available at: http://www.scielo.cl/scielo.php?script=sci_arttext&pid=S0034-98872013000800013&lng=es. Accessed Ago 16, 2017.

10. Montero X, San Martín J, Cohen M, et al. Audiological evaluation of children with autism in developing countries. Otolaryngol Head Neck Surg 2004;131(2):A1–40. P1-P360.

11. Wong L-Y, Espinoza F, Mojica K, et al. Otoacoustic emissions in rural Nicaragua: cost analysis and implications for newborn hearing screening. Otolaryngol Head Neck Surg 2017;156(5):877–85. Available at: http://otojournal.org. Accessed August 16, 2017.

12. Chiossone E. Current status of cochlear implants in Latin America. Am J Otol 1995;16(2):183–5.

13. Goycoolea MV, Latin American Cochlear Implant Group. Latin American experience with the cochlear implant. Acta Otolaryngol 2005;125(5):468–73.

14. Armengol K. Mexico: exponential advances in cochlear implants. 2014. Available at: http://www.audiology-worldnews.com/focus-on/941-mexico-exponential-advances-in-cochlear-implants. Accessed August 29, 2017.

15. Federación AICE. El implante coclear en Latinoamérica. 2013. Available at: http://federacionaice.implantecoclear.org/index.php/articulos-archivados/96-news/latest-news/269-el-implante-coclear-en-latinoamerica. Accessed August 16, 2017.

16. Curado MP, Johnson NW, Kerr AR, et al. Oral and oropharynx cancer in South America: incidence, mortality trends and gaps in public databases as presented to the Global Oral Cancer Forum. Translational Res Oral Oncol 2016;1:1–7.

17. Warnakulasuriya S. Global epidemiology of oral and oropharyngeal cancer. Oral Oncol 2009;45:309–16.

18. Curado MP, Hashibe M. Recent changes in the epidemiology of head and neck cancer. Curr Opin Oncol 2009;21:194–200.

19. Wyss A, Hashibe M, Chuang SC, et al. Cigarette, cigar, and pipe smoking and the risk of head and neck cancers: pooled analysis in the International Head and Neck Cancer Epidemiology Consortium. Am J Epidemiol 2013;178(5):679–90.

20. Bruni L, Barrionuevo-Rosas L, Albero G, et al. Human papillomavirus and related diseases in the world. Summary report: July 27, 2017. Barcelona (Spain): ICO/IARC Information Centre on HPV and Cancer; 2017.

21. Goldenberg D, Golz A, Joachims HZ. The beverage maté: a risk factor for cancer of the head and neck. Head Neck 2003;25(7):595–601.

22. Loria D, Barrios E, Zanetti R. Cancer and yerba mate consumption: a review of possible associations. Rev Panam Salud Publica 2009;25(6):530–9.

23. UNAIDS. The prevention gap report. 2016. Available at: http://www.unaids.org/sites/default/files/media_asset/2016-prevention-gap-report_en.pdf. Accessed August 29, 2017.

24. Children and HIV/AIDS in Latin America and the Caribbean, Challenges: UNICEF newsletter, number 7, July 2008.

25. Jimenez MA, Cabrera J, Fiol JJ, et al. Antiretroviral treatment in the spotlight: a public health analysis in Latin America and the Caribbean 2013. Washington, DC: PAHO; 2013. ISBN 978-92-75-11806-1.

26. Prasad HK, Bhojwani KM, Shenoy V, et al. HIV manifestations in otolaryngology. Am J Otolaryngol 2006;27(3):179–85.

27. Ranganathan K, Hemalatha R. Oral lesions in HIV infection in developing countries: an overview. Adv Dent Res 2006;19(1):63–8.

Workforce Considerations, Training, and Diseases of the Asia-Pacific Region

James D. Smith, MD[a,b],*, Keng Lu Tan, MD[c]

KEYWORDS

- Asia • Otolaryngology • Workforce • Residency training • Diseases

KEY POINTS

- The Asia-Pacific region is the largest and most diverse region in the world and contains 60% of the world's population.
- The otolaryngology workforce varies depending on the number of doctors in the country, the scope of practice, and availability of posttraining employment.
- Otolaryngology training has been influenced by the British, Russian, and US training systems.
- A common weakness of otolaryngology is the lack of hands-on surgical training.
- Otolaryngologic diseases in the Asia-Pacific region are similar to those seen in the United States but with many ethnic and regional differences.

INTRODUCTION

The Asia-Pacific region is the largest and most diverse region discussed in this issue. It includes most of Russia, most of the countries of the former Soviet Union, China, Japan, North and South Korea, India, 10 Association of Southeast Asian Nations countries, Australia, and New Zealand, as well as several other smaller countries. These countries contain 60% of the world's population, a total of 4.6 billion people. Health care resources vary from high-income countries (eg, Japan, Australia, New Zealand, Hong Kong, and Singapore) to low-income countries (eg, Nepal and North Korea) and, in between, middle-income countries (eg, Russia, China, and India). It is not possible to cover global health specifics in any detail for such a diverse population;

Disclosure Statement: The authors have nothing to disclose.
[a] Department of Otolaryngology, Oregon Health & Science University, 3181 SW Sam Jackson Park Road, Portland, OR 97239, USA; [b] Department of Otolaryngology, National University of Singapore, 1E Kent Ridge Road, NUHS Tower Block, Level 11, Singapore 119228; [c] Department of Otolaryngology, Ipoh Specialist Hospital, 30, Jalan Raja Dihilir, Ipoh, Perak 30350, Malaysia
* Corresponding author. 16124 Northwest St. Andrews Drive, Portland, OR 97229.
E-mail address: jamesd.smith@yahoo.com

Otolaryngol Clin N Am 51 (2018) 659–665
https://doi.org/10.1016/j.otc.2018.01.010
0030-6665/18/© 2018 Elsevier Inc. All rights reserved.

however, this article discusses general concepts about otolaryngology health care in the region.

POPULATIONS

The Asia-Pacific region includes the 2 most populous countries in the world: China with 1.5 billion and India with 1.3 billion, as well as many other countries and ethnic groups. With such a huge geographic area and different ethnic groups, the health problems are equally diverse. As an example, until recently, most global drug studies had been carried out in Western Europe and North America. Although there can be a difference in the metabolism or effectiveness of certain drugs in different ethnic populations, there are relatively few studies looking at the efficacy of drugs in varying ethnic groups.[1]

WORKFORCE CONSIDERATIONS

In Asia, as elsewhere, low-income countries and, to a lesser extent, middle-income countries have a relatively small health care workforce available per population compared with high-income countries. It may be assumed that the otolaryngology workforce would mirror that of all physicians; however, numbers are difficult to find in the literature. The International Federation of Oto-Rhino-Laryngological Societies (IFOS) has a listing of the number of otolaryngologists for many countries; however, it may not accurately represent the total for some countries because it may only include otolaryngology society members in the country instead of all practicing otolaryngologists (**Table 1**).[2] There are many potential reasons for the discrepancy in the number of otolaryngologists per country. Too few medical graduates, poor salaries, or lack of interest in otolaryngology. Also, historically, many medical graduates, including otolaryngologists, have emigrated from Asia to Europe and North America.

When comparing workforce needs for otolaryngology, the scope of practice must also be considered. The United States arguably has the broadest scope of otolaryngology practice anywhere in the world. The scope of otolaryngology practice in Asia

Table 1 Population per otolaryngologist for 12 countries in Asia			
Country	Population in Millions	Otolaryngologists	Otolaryngologist per Population
China	1500	20,000	1:40,600[a]
India	1324	5768	1:229,542[17]
Indonesia	261.1	1374	1:190,000[2]
Pakistan	193.2	90	1:2.146 million[2]
Bangladesh	163	90	1:1.811 million[2]
Russia	144.3	Unknown	Unknown[2]
Japan	127	4080	1:31,000[2]
Philippines	103.3	865	1:119,421[18]
Vietnam	92.7	70	1:1.322 million[2]
Thailand	68.7	1300	1:53,000[2]
Malaysia	31.2	400	1:78,000[2]
Taiwan	23.55	2600	1:9057[2]

[a] Estimated because statistics combine otolaryngology with ophthalmology because there are still doctors who practice both specialties in more rural areas. The number used here for otolaryngology was 50% of the total.

depends more on the abilities of the surgeon and the facilities available. For example, the rhinologists in Myanmar are not able to practice what they learn in the United States because they do not have the instruments and endoscopy equipment that were available where they trained. In Singapore, the scope of practice does not include as much facial plastics, and the general otolaryngologist does relatively fewer tonsillectomy and adenoidectomies or myringotomies with ventilation tubes. Many countries in the Asia-Pacific region are moving toward subspecialty practices. Although in some countries the subspecialties are not clearly carved out, the patients and general physicians prefer otolaryngology–head and neck surgeons to manage head and neck diseases. In other countries, such as China, only otolaryngologists in an academic or government hospital do major surgical procedures. Even in major teaching hospitals, local rules or training may dictate which procedures are done. When evaluating the otolaryngology workforce, the number of residents trained, the scope of practice, and adequate compensation on completion of the training program must be considered. Balancing the production of otolaryngologists and need is a delicate and imprecise science for all countries.

China has a unique aspect of their workforce in Traditional Chinese Medicine (TCM), which is an integral part of the medical community. Otolaryngologists working in Asia should have at least a tacit knowledge of TCM. TCM is a specific alternative health care practice that is common in China and many other Asian countries. TCM is widely practiced in other regions of the Pacific, with variations that sometimes may resemble myth more than science. Examples include Ayurveda in India and Jamu in Polynesian countries. In China alone, the TCM sector provided care for 7 million inpatients and 200 million outpatients in 2006, or 10% to 20% of all Chinese health care.[3] A recent study from Taiwan found that 29% of chronic rhinosinusitis patients used TCM in addition to Western medicine.[4] The number of practitioners and hospitals in China offering TCM has increased in recent years.[5]

The origins of TCM date back to the third century BC. The principles of TCM involve concepts of balance between the opposite energies of Yin and Yang, as well as the life force, Chi. Treatment in TCM consists of herbal remedies, acupuncture, food therapy, massage, and exercise. Although TCM focuses on herbal medicines and holistic management of patients, in contrast to the more molecular focus of Western medicine on disease, proponents of the scientific basis for TCM claim that the beneficial effects stem from alterations in agonist and antagonist action of neurotransmitters such as dopamine and serotonin.

Some TCM treatments for otolaryngology diseases include those for otitis media, allergic rhinitis, chronic rhinosinusitis, and tinnitus. Otitis media treatments include a variety of herbal medicines, acupuncture, and Qigong (Chinese breathing exercise). Similarly, herbal therapy is a commonly recommended TCM for treatment of chronic rhinosinusitis, with Bai Zhi the most commonly used single herb. A wide variety of alternative treatments have been used to treat tinnitus, including acupuncture and *Gingko biloba*. The effectiveness of these treatments is unproven.

The use of TCM may delay patients in seeking care from physicians using Western medicine. In addition, some TCM treatments have been associated with adverse reactions. These potential adverse reactions include heavy metal contamination, bleeding dyscrasias, cardiotoxicity, nephrotoxicity, or carcinogenicity. Otolaryngologists are most likely to encounter these toxicities in the management of epistaxis. The TCM herbal treatments *Ginkgo biloba*, Chinese angelica (*Angelica sinensis*), and *Salvia miltiorrhiza* may all lead to severe bleeding problems.[3] Dr Sam Rosen was the first recorded American otolaryngologist to visit China after the Cultural Revolution, observing the Chinese experience using acupuncture to treat sensorineural hearing loss. In 1974, he reported his personal disappointing experience in using acupuncture to treat children with sensorineural hearing loss in the United States at the American Laryngology, Rhinology, and Otology Society meeting.[6]

TRAINING

Residency training in such a diverse group of countries is as varied as the countries represented. The British-style training program sponsored by the 4 Royal Colleges of Surgeons in the United Kingdom has a direct influence on former members of the British Empire. This is true in India, Pakistan, Australia, New Zealand, Hong Kong, Malaysia, and Singapore. Until about 2001, many otolaryngology residents from Asian countries would go to the United Kingdom, especially Edinburgh, to take the Fellowship of the Royal College of Surgeons (FRCS) examination and return home as consultants or enter advanced surgical (otolaryngology) training. Some countries have made their own modifications for a local otolaryngology exit (board) examination, with their own standards. In most countries, a specialist must have some type of recognized posttraining examination to be listed on the Ministry of Health registry of specialists, a necessary requirement to practice a specialty.

Currently, training programs for otolaryngology within the region are also open for fellowship training of doctors from other countries. As an example, Bhutanese and Nepalese have trained in Malaysia and other nearby countries. Some of the qualifications need to be verified on return to their respective countries, while others are cross-recognized. Until now, many of the specialists in the Asia-Pacific region were trained in the United Kingdom or United States. Their qualifications are recognized in most Asian countries; however, usually those able to take advantage of these opportunities are those with personal finances or government sponsorship.

Accreditation Council for Graduate Medical Education (ACGME) formed ACGME-International (ACGME-I) to offer their expertise in residency training to overseas countries for a fee. The Singapore Ministry of Health was the first country to take advantage of this offer and did a major restructuring of all of their residency training programs, including otolaryngology.[7] There was also the hope that specialty boards from the American Board of Medical Specialties (ABMS) would make their board examinations available to Singapore residents to take the place of the FRCS examination. Each ABMS specialty has made different agreements; however, the American Board of Otolaryngology (ABO) helped by sharing some of their multiple choice questions, helping local otolaryngologists develop questions locally, and sending an external examiner for the oral examination. Locally, it was hoped that the ABO would make a separate certification called a Fellow of the ABO-International. In this way, the local examination would have some type of international recognition similar to the old FRCS. However, that was not ultimately approved by the ABO.

Understanding residency training in China continues to be challenging. At present, medical school is for 5 years after high school for most students. Everyone has to take a national examination that qualifies them for licensure. In the past, there were 2 tracks: academic, leading to a master's and/or a PhD, and the other a clinical track. The academic track had an emphasis on research and limited clinical experience. Currently, there is still the degree path; however, most doctors in both tracks are required to do a 2-year to 3-year residency (stage I). The government mandates required rotations; however, residents often spend less than 25% of their time in their chosen specialty, such as otolaryngology. This leaves them poorly equipped to practice the specialty independently and, therefore, most residents stay for another 2 to 3 years at the hospital that hired them and do a stage II residency to gain enough experience to become independent. Each hospital, university, prefect, or city will determine when the resident is qualified to practice because there are no national standards such as from the ABMS or from specialty boards such as the ABO.[8]

For Russia and the former Soviet Union countries, the Russian style training is predominant.[9] In some other countries in Asia, the type and quality of training, is variable. Two main problems are a tendency for learning by rote memory rather than application and a lack of hands-on surgical experience. In many countries the lack of hands-on experience is balanced by a long period of time as a trainee or junior faculty member. This will often lead to subspecialists in the universities or major hospitals. Those outside these systems are left to do only minor surgical procedures and medical otolaryngology. As a result, the quality of otolaryngology care can be quite variable.

OTOLARYNGOLOGIC DISEASES

Diseases treated by otolaryngologists in Asia are similar to those seen in the Western world; however, with significant differences. The Chinese population of Southeast Asia has the world's highest prevalence of undifferentiated carcinoma of the nasopharynx, whereas in North America the prevalence is several factors less.[10] In multiracial countries such as Malaysia, diseases are stratified by race. Nasopharyngeal carcinoma is seen most commonly among Chinese, followed by Malays, and almost nonexistent in southern Indians.[11] Lop ear is very common; however, it is not generally bothersome to the Malays, and some Chinese believe that lop ears signify good hearing. A deviated nasal septum with external deformities affects the Punjab Indians more than other races. In India, there is a high incidence of profound hearing loss from congenital and acquired etiologic factors. Because the government has recognized this problem, there have been almost 200 state-of-the-art cochlear implant centers established across India over the last few years to meet this need.[12] In India and other South East Asian countries, the practice of chewing betel nut is a major etiologic agent for oral squamous cell carcinoma.[13] In Singapore, perennial allergic rhinitis caused by house dust mites is a major part of an otolaryngologist's practice. In tropical areas there is a higher incidence of malaria and tuberculosis. Human immunodeficiency virus–AIDS is a problem in several Asian countries. In many countries, the spread is through the sex trade, especially in Thailand, Myanmar, and Indonesia. In some cases, it is spread by contaminated needles from either intravenous drug use or is iatrogenic. In other cases, it may be from contaminated blood supplies.[14] The diverse Asian population highlights the importance of conducting disease prevalence studies and drug studies across a wide population of diverse ethnic groups.

Vehicular trauma is very high in many of these countries. Diseases such as sleep apnea and gastroesophageal reflux disease are relatively common, despite most people not being overweight.[15] Other common problems, especially in China, are foreign body aspiration in children and cleft lip or palate. Probably the greatest difference between Asia and the United States is not the disease but the variability of who treats specific diseases.

OPPORTUNITIES FOR HUMANITARIAN SERVICE

There are many opportunities for short-term medical volunteer trips in low-income countries and middle-income countries in the Asian region. Individuals or groups looking for humanitarian opportunities should try to work with national otolaryngologists clinically and/or in an academic setting, especially to share experiences and training. This will allow the most sustainable long-term results with the possibility of changing the future of otolaryngology in any given country. One of the best examples of this is the long-term relationships developed in Vietnam over the past 20 years by a group of otolaryngologists from the American Academy of Otolaryngology who have made biannual visits. With ongoing reciprocal visits, the level of otolaryngology training and patient care has improved in Vietnam.[16]

SUMMARY

Considering that 60% of the world's population lives in the Asia-Pacific region, it is not surprising there are differences in workforce needs, training, and otolaryngologic diseases. As with otolaryngology in the United States, otolaryngology in Asia is constantly changing and improving. The differences in care are fascinating and should lead otolaryngologists to continue to share experiences and training, ultimately leading to better global patient care.

REFERENCES

1. Gevaert P, Van Bruaene N, Cattaret T, et al. Mepolizumab, a humanized anti-IL-5 mAb as a treatment option for severe nasal polyps. J Allergy Clin Immunol 2011; 128:989–95.
2. Website: list of IFOS members. Available at: http://www.ifosworld.org/members. php. Accessed July 24, 2017.
3. Tang JL, Liu BY, Ma KW. Traditional Chinese medicine. Lancet 2008;372(9654): 1938–40.
4. Yen HR, Sun MF, Lin CL, et al. Adjunctive traditional Chinese medicine therapy for patients with chronic rhinosinusitis: a population-based study. Int Forum Allergy Rhinol 2015;5(3):240–6.
5. Health care with Chinese characteristics: why China's traditional medicine boom is dangerous. The Economist 2017.
6. Rosen S. Feasibility of acupuncture as a treatment for sensori-neural deafness in children. Laryngoscope 1974;84:2202–17.
7. Website: ACGME-I History. Available at: http://www.acgme-i.org/About-Us/ History. Accessed July 25, 2017.
8. Wu L, Wang Y, Peng X, et al. Development of a medical academic degree system in China. Med Educ Online 2014;19:23141.
9. Jargin SV. Some aspects of medical education in Russia. American Journal of Medicine Studies 2013;1(2):4–7.
10. Cao S, Simons MJ, Qian C. The prevalence and prevention of nasopharyngeal carcinoma in China. Chin J Cancer 2011;30(2):114–9.
11. Aziz A, Ramli R, Mohamad I, et al. Young nasopharyngeal carcinoma: a review of an 8-year experience in the East Coast Malaysia Hospital. The Egyptian Journal of Otolaryngology 2017;33(2):490–4.
12. Kumar RNS, Kameswaran M. Cochlear implantation in the developing world: perspectives from the Indian subcontinent. ENT Audiol News 2017;26(4):88–9.
13. Anand R, Dhingra C, Prasad S, et al. Betel nut chewing and its deleterious effects on oral cavity. J Cancer Res Ther 2014;10(3):499–505.
14. Website: HIV and AIDS in Asia & the pacific regional overview. Available at: https://www.avert.org/professionals/hiv-around-world/asia-pacific/overview. Accessed July 26, 2017.
15. Lam B, Lam DC, Ip MS. Obstructive sleep apnoea in Asia. Int J Tuberc Lung Dis 2007;11(1):2–11.
16. Bailey BJ. Medical missions to Vietnam and Cuba: lessons in global education. Laryngoscope 2007;117(10):1703–9.

17. Association of Otolaryngologists India (AOI). Registered Number of ENT Surgeons in India. Springer. Available at: http://aoiho.org/pages/views/memberslist. Accessed July 31, 2017.

18. Philippine Society of Otolaryngology–Head and Neck Surgery. About us. PSO-HNS. Available at: http://pso-hns.org/about-us/#our-story. Accessed July 31, 2017.

Workforce Considerations, Training, and Diseases in the Middle East

George Richard Holt, MD, MSE, MPH, MABE, D Bioethics[a],*,
Kevin Christopher McMains, MD[b], Randal A. Otto, MD[a]

KEYWORDS

- Middle East otolaryngology • Global health in the Middle East
- Disease prevalence in the Middle East
- Medical education and training in otolaryngology in the Middle East

KEY POINTS

- Prevalent diseases in the Middle East include the noncommunicable diseases of coronary artery disease, stroke, diabetes, and head and neck cancer (the latter due to the high rates of tobacco usage).
- Health care system capabilities range from struggling economies to high sophistication in developed countries.
- War, conflict, strife, and government instability give rise to great challenges in providing adequate health care in some countries of the Middle East.
- Medical education and training in otolaryngology was previously based on the European system but increasing incorporation of the American system is occurring.
- In some countries, there is great personal risk to physicians caring for patients and to visiting physicians from other countries.

INTRODUCTION AND OVERVIEW OF HEALTH STATUS AND DISEASES IN THE MIDDLE EAST

The Middle East is a complex area of the world, not only demographically but also in the diverse governmental, political, social, religious, financial, and medical contexts. In general, the Middle East is a group of 18 countries in the eastern Mediterranean and Persian Gulf, which includes Egypt in North Africa and Palestine. Turkey and Cyprus

Disclosure: The authors have nothing to disclose.
[a] Department of Otolaryngology–Head and Neck Surgery, The University of Texas Health Science Center, Mail Code 7777, 8300 Floyd Curl Drive, San Antonio, TX 78229, USA; [b] Division of Otolaryngology–Head and Neck Surgery, Audie Murphy Veterans Administration Medical Center, 7400 Merton Minter Street, San Antonio, TX 78229, USA
* Corresponding author.
E-mail address: holtg@uthscsa.edu

Otolaryngol Clin N Am 51 (2018) 667–673
https://doi.org/10.1016/j.otc.2018.01.011
0030-6665/18/© 2018 Elsevier Inc. All rights reserved.

oto.theclinics.com

may be included in discussions of Middle Eastern countries but not always. The US Department of State's Bureau of Near Eastern Affairs includes the following countries, states, or territory in their purview: Palestinian territories, Qatar, Saudi Arabia, Syria, Tunisia, United Arab Emirates, Algeria, Bahrain, Egypt, Iran, Iraq, Israel, Jordan, Kuwait, Lebanon, Libya, Morocco, Oman, and Yemen.[1] Additionally, the League of Arab States has 22 members, and is a cooperative and functional unit acting in the Middle East.

Germane to the health care systems of these countries, several governmental models exist. There are 3 constitutional monarchies (Qatar, Kuwait, and Bahrain), 2 absolute monarchies (Saudi Arabia and Oman), 1 federal monarchy (United Arab Emirates), 1 parliamentary democracy (Israel), 1 theocratic republic (Iran), 1 presidential republic (Syria), 1 parliamentary monarchy (Jordan), and other federal government models of various governments. Thus, there is a broad range of financial capabilities to support effective health care delivery and to develop and sustain an infrastructure for each country's health care system. Language and religious variances within each country and between countries challenges cooperative efforts in health care delivery.

Unlike Europe and the Far East, many countries in the Middle East are, and have been for some time, in a constant state of conflict and combat. The Middle East is the epicenter of global terrorism, and countries such as Iraq, Afghanistan, and Syria have such a burden of trauma cases that limited medical resources are often stretched beyond their limits. Basic services may be minimal, and preventive health in many regions is nonexistent. There are significant challenges to the delivery of health care in hostile and intemperate geographic terrains from desert to mountains. Rural health care in isolated parts of some countries is often rudimentary, provided only by marginally trained lower level health care workers who do the best they can with minimal resources and limited higher echelon support.

Emerging medical services may lack the sophistication and robustness of Western medicine, especially in ambulance and first-responder capabilities. Trauma patients (especially from terrorist attacks) are often transported to a hospital by passing motorists or bystanders. Triage and emergency care resources are often limited to basic life-saving treatments, and tertiary or specialized care centers are often few and far between. Trauma care is becoming a priority for otolaryngology in the Middle East, driven by injuries due to war and terrorism. Both intrinsic and foreign teaching in the management of head and neck trauma is increasing in training programs across this region.

Alternatively, several countries in the Middle East (eg, Saudi Arabia, United Arab Emirates, Jordan, Israel, Turkey, and Qatar) have quite sophisticated and modern health care systems, typically based on the British system of education and training of physicians and nurses. Resources are plentiful and funding is relatively generous. Medical education and specialty training can be comparable to that of Western medicine, including tertiary academic medical centers where meaningful research is conducted, and the full range of specialty care is provided.

General Health Conditions

Using data from the Global Burden of Diseases, Injuries, and Risk Factor Studies (GBD), heart disease was the number 1 cause of death in the Arab world in 2010, replacing lower respiratory diseases.[2] Risk factors for death included processed foods, hypertension, high body-mass index, diabetes, and hypercholesterolemia. Major depressive disorder, especially in women, and lower back pain, in men, contributed to higher years lived with disability in most of these countries. Road injuries and other occupational risks are more common in those more highly developed countries where transportation and driving are reflective of a more robust economy. Communicable diseases, such as malaria and diarrhea, still have a concerning prevalence but new public health concerns include noncommunicable diseases, with respect to lifestyle changes.[3] There is concern that the Middle East region "suffers a drastic change from a traditional diet to an industrialized diet,"[4] with the attendant increase in chronic diseases affected by the ingestion of increased preprocessed foods, sugar, and saturated fats, with a reduction of healthier milk, fruits, and vegetables. The long-term effects of these dietary changes on the genome are not yet fully appreciated, but chronic disease prevalence may already be affected.

Communicable and Respiratory Diseases

Additional communicable diseases include hepatitis, human immunodeficiency virus, and the Middle East respiratory syndrome. Of considerable concern to the World Health Organization is that the prevalence of hepatitis C in the Middle East is high, with Egypt reportedly experiencing the highest rate of hepatitis C in the world.[5] This rate may exceed 10%, with inadequate infection control and unscreened blood transfusions as major factors.

Middle East respiratory syndrome is an acute illness caused by the virus Middle East respiratory syndrome coronavirus (MERS-CoV). First reported in Saudi Arabia in 2012, it is said to be unlike other coronaviruses previously found in humans.[6] This respiratory disease is of concern because of the 30% to 40% fatality rate associated with outbreaks. US health care providers traveling to the Arabian Peninsula should maintain a high level of awareness and use personal protective equipment in areas of risk.

There are other respiratory disorders of concern in the Middle East, and they carry a health burden for the population and health care delivery systems: tuberculosis; bacterial, viral, parasitic, and fungal pneumonias; Behçet disease; and complications of chemical warfare. Unique aspects related to respiratory diseases in the Middle East include climate factors in the desert region, cultural habits, and water-pipe smoking, as well as heavy cigarette use.[7]

Head and Neck Cancer

With the high prevalence of smoking, head and neck cancer incidence is increasing. In areas where the health care system is sophisticated, the full range of head and neck cancer therapy is available; otherwise, limitations in cancer care are predictable. There are increasingly positive trends, however, in comprehensive head and neck cancer care, owing in part to broader clinical and educational collaborations among Middle East countries, and with Europe, North America, and international agencies. Furtherance of these collaborations should be a salutary goal of global otolaryngology–head and neck surgery organizations.

High rates of head and neck cancer, particularly oral cavity and oropharynx carcinomas, in the Middle East are due to smoking and chewing tobacco. In a recent epidemiologic report, the prevalence of tobacco smoking in the Middle East and North Africa in male patients over the age of 15 years varies from a low of 15% in Oman to a high of 77% in Yemen, with most other countries in the 30% to 60% range.[8] Female patients were noted to have one-tenth the rate of smoking compared with men. The authors, using established predictions, project that the number of estimated new cases of oral and oropharynx cancers in this region, especially in Egypt, Iran, and Turkey, could double by the year 2030, 4 times the predicted incidence worldwide. A swell in the aging population in these countries (ie, living longer) may be a factor.[9] Reducing high-risk factors such as smoking and use of smokeless tobacco (shammah and qat), and perhaps exploring or mitigating the risks for human papilloma virus infections, could be effective public health methods to address this projected increase in cancer incidence.[10]

In a report of the Middle East Cancer Consortium (MECC), thyroid cancer contributes 1.5% to 3.80% of all cancers diagnosed annually in the 4 MECC countries studied (Cyprus, Egypt, Israel, and Jordan).[11] Female patients in the regions were found to have twice the incidence of thyroid cancers compared with male patients. Age-standardized incidence rates across the countries ranged from 2.0 in Egypt to 7.5 in Israeli Jews. Egypt, in particular, has a very high incidence of anaplastic thyroid cancer (14%) compared with the other MECC countries and the United States (<3%). Egypt also showed the lowest rate of differentiated thyroid carcinomas (73%) than the other 3 MECC countries studied (90%–94%).[11]

The MECC report also addressed laryngeal carcinomas in the 4 countries studied. Age-standardized incidence rates for laryngeal carcinoma in Israeli Jews, Jordanians, and Egyptians were found to be commensurate with the US Surveillance, Epidemiology, and End Results (SEER) program rates. However, the rate in Israeli Arab male patients (6.0) was higher than comparable US SEER male patients (4.6).[12] The incidence of laryngeal cancer in female patients in the studied populations was quite low. Because alcohol consumption is considered to be minimal in predominately Muslim Middle Eastern countries, the epidemiologic preventative focus is being placed on reducing smoking in the at-risk populations.

WORKFORCE, EDUCATION, AND TRAINING IN OTOLARYNGOLOGY–HEAD AND NECK SURGERY IN THE MIDDLE EAST

The modern Middle East represents a vital and varied combination of ancient and ultramodern, densely populated and vast spaces, of countries and cultures influencing and being influenced by the cultural and economic effects of globalization while honoring tradition. This is as true in medicine as it is in other fields. Traditions of medical education and practice are both long and proud in the region. From Avicenna through Maimonides and beyond, contributions of physicians and surgeons from this region have both preserved and advanced the understanding of medicine and of the philosophic implications if its practice.

It is impossible to fully understand the modern medical systems in the varied countries of the region without delving into a bit of history. During World War I, the Ottoman Empire entered the conflict on the side of the Central Powers: Germany and the Austro-Hungarian Empire. As the war concluded, several European powers maintained colonial empires, even as the Ottoman Empire dissolved. Much can be written about the ethics of empire and governance of people and cultures by outside powers, though that is beyond the scope of this article. One product of European influence in the Middle East was the Sykes-Picot Agreement.[13] In this agreement, the Triple Entente (England, France, and Russia) agreed to separate spheres of influence within what was then called Asia-Minor, without significant consideration of local cultures and populations. The resulting English mandate would govern much of modern Iraq, Jordan, and modern Israel, whereas the French mandate would govern northern Iraq, Syria, Lebanon, and eastern Turkey. The national boundaries later established in the region largely ignored cultural, tribal, and sectarian affiliations, setting the stage for much of the conflict resulting in this region in the subsequent century.

The university level educational systems established in the region were largely modeled on those present in the country claiming mandate within that geography. With increasing American influence in the region following World War II, there has been a growing acceptance of the American medical educational model as well. As countries in the region sought to speed modernization, many made university education available at low or no cost. Because of the prestige of a medical degree, there is considerable familial and societal pressure for students to select medicine, which is an undergraduate course of study in the British system (A. Atef, personal communication, 2017). Resulting rates of medical degree holders range widely from 0.311 per 1000 population in Yemen to 3.62 per 1000 in Israel. This compares with 2.55 in the US and 2.48 in Canada.[14]

Although several countries within the region boast impressive Graduate Medical Education opportunities, countries may lack a coordinated national health policy that aligns undergraduate and graduate medical education.[15] Therefore, many trainees elect to receive training outside the region. This is true of otolaryngology, as it is for other medical and surgical specialties. As early as 1994, articles appeared encouraging an increase in graduate-level otolaryngology training within the Arab world.[16] One limitation to surgical training is inherited traditions that prohibit cadaveric dissection (A. Atef, personal communication, 2017). In recent years, simulation has been used to bridge this gap.[17] Another confounding issue with practice is that no single standard for credentialing exists. Whereas many countries recognize the Arab Boards, many recognize local boards, PhD degrees, and certifying examinations from Europe, England, or America.

Two major challenges to delivery of high-quality otolaryngology care throughout the Middle East are large populations and political instability. Although this affords trainees a wealth of training opportunity, demand for otolaryngology services far outstrips the supply available in many communities. In such situations, regional academic otolaryngology faculty members often care for the flood of patients with extremely advanced disease. Faculty members working in these centers are forced to be creative to meet specific surgical challenges and system demands. In recent years, both armed conflict and political change following the Arab Spring uprising have increased challenges to providing effective graduate and continuing medical education in many Middle Eastern Countries. Not only has funding for medical centers and faculty been threatened and inconsistent but also, for a time, outside speakers were reluctant to participate in regional conferences because of personal security concerns. Tightening borders in Europe and the United States increases challenges to otolaryngologists who would otherwise attend conferences in these regions. Especially needed in the Middle East are more female otolaryngologists, reflective of the general requirement for female physicians across the world but especially in the male-dominant Middle East medical profession; however, advances are being made to better reflect Western gender balances in specialty training.

Potential solutions to these problems are many. Regional educational conferences continue to showcase both the vast surgical skills within the region and an equally vast desire to continue to advance practice. These conferences are attended by otolaryngologists from the Middle East and the West alike. Professional organizations such as the American Academy of Otolaryngology–Head and Neck Surgery and Foundation continue to work toward increasing access to high-quality educational opportunities through sponsoring of joint meetings, travel grants and scholarships, and International Corresponding Society relationships. In those regions with high-speed Internet access, platforms for delivery of synchronous and asynchronous educational content will continue to expand and improve the ability of otolaryngologists throughout the Middle East to participate in training opportunities without the requirements of travel.

In a region justly proud of its culture and contributions to medicine, the ingenuity and drive of otolaryngologists to continue to teach and to create opportunity for their own advancement will certainly meet the present challenges.

SUMMARY

The challenges for health care delivery in Middle Eastern countries are many, varied, and complex. Chronic diseases are on the increase and there is a high burden of disease, especially with pulmonary infections, head and neck cancers, and trauma, for which assistance from international organizations and professionals is needed. It must be emphasized, however, that even in the face of constant strife and conflict and very limited resources in some countries, the dedication of health care providers is exemplary. These professionals, including otolaryngologist surgeons, care for patients under often dangerous conditions and continue to do so in the face of their own potential peril. This dedication is worthy of praise and recognition.

REFERENCES

1. US Department of State. Bureau of Near Eastern Affairs. Available at: https://www.state.gov/p/nea/. Accessed September 12, 2017.
2. Mokdad AH, Jaber S, Aziz MI, et al. The state of health in the Arab world, 1990–2010: an analysis of the burden of diseases, injuries, and risk factors. Lancet 2014;383(9914):309–20.
3. World Health Organization. Regional office for the Eastern Mediterranean. Framework for health information systems and core indicators for monitoring health situation and health system performance. 2016. Available at: https://applications.emro.who.int/dsaf/EMROPUB_2016_EN_19169.pdf?ua=1. Accessed September 8, 2017.
4. Fahed AC, El-Hage-Sleiman AKM, Farhat TI, et al. Diet, genetics, and disease: a focus on the Middle East and North Africa region. J Nutr Metab 2012. https://doi.org/10.1155/2012/109037.
5. Averhoff FM, Glass N, Holtzman D. Global burden of hepatitis C: considerations for healthcare providers in the United States. Clin Infect Dis 2012;55(Suppl 1):S10–5.
6. Department of Health and Human Services. Centers for Disease Control and Prevention. Information about Middle East Respiratory Syndrome (MERS). 2015. Available at: https://www.cdc.gov/coronavirus/mers/about/index.html. Accessed September 22, 2017.
7. Waness A, El-Sameed YA, Mahboub B, et al. Respiratory disorders in the Middle East: a review. Respirology 2011;16:755–66.
8. Kujan O, Farah CS, Johnson NW. Oral and oropharyngeal cancer in the Middle East and North Africa: incidence mortality, trends, and gaps in public databases as presented to the Global Oral Cancer Forum. Translational Research in Oral Oncology 2017;2:1–9.
9. Hajjar RR, Atli T, Al-Mandhari Z, et al. Prevalence of aging population in the Middle East and its implications on cancer incidence and care. Ann Oncol 2013;24(Suppl):vii11–24.
10. Al-Jaber A, Al-Nasser L, El-Metwally A. Epidemiology of oral cancer in Arab countries. Saudi Med J 2016;37:249–55.
11. Ronckers C, Ron E. Thyroid cancer. Chapter 13. In: Freedman LS, Edwards BK, Ries LAG, et al, editors. Cancer incidence in four member countries (Cyprus, Egypt, Israel, and Jordan) of the Middle East Cancer Consortium (MECC) compared with US SEER. Bethesda (MD): National Cancer Institute; 2006. p. 121–9.
12. Al-Kayed S, Qasem MB. Laryngeal cancer. Chapter 7. In: Freedman LS, Edwards BK, Ries LAG, et al, editors. Cancer incidence in four member countries (Cyprus, Egypt, Israel, and Jordan) of the Middle East Cancer Consortium

(MECC) compared with US SEER. Bethesda (MD): National Cancer Institute; 2006. p. 69–72.

13. Anderson S. Lawrence in Arabia: war, deceit, imperial folly and the making of the modern Middle East. New York: Random House; 2014.

14. Density of physicians (total number per 1000 population, latest available year) Global Health Observatory (GHO) data. Geneva (Switzerland): World Health Organization; 2017. Available at: http://www.who.int/gho/health_workforce/physicians_density/en/.

15. Schoenbaum SC, Crome P, Curry RH, et al. Policy issues related to educating the future Israeli medical workforce: an international perspective. Isr J Health Policy Res 2015;4:37.

16. Baraka ME. Medical education: an audit of an overseas postgraduate training programme in ENT. J Laryngol Otol 1994;108(12):1072–5.

17. Abou-Elhamd KE, Al-Sultan AI, Rashad UM. Simulation in ENT medical education. J Laryngol Otol 2010;124(3):237–41.

Workforce Considerations, Training, and Certification of Physicians in Europe

Maria V. Suurna, MD[a,*], Eugene N. Myers, MD[b], Sebastian Roesch, MD[c]

KEYWORDS

- Health care • Health insurance • Physician training • Medical education
- Certification

KEY POINTS

- Europe is confronted with the issue of lack of health care access and workforce shortage.
- Geopolitical events, aging population, nonstandardized medical training, and mobility of health care professionals influence the current state of health care in the European Union (EU).
- There is a need to develop unified health care programs, standardized medical training, and certification across the EU countries to address uneven access and quality of health care, as well as workforce shortage.

INTRODUCTION

Workforce considerations, physician training, and certification in Europe have never been more important. The geopolitical events in the twentieth century included 2 World Wars and nearly a half century of Communist domination of large parts of Europe. These events may not have caused as much sociopolitical upheaval as the enormous population shifts of the twenty-first century caused by the migration to Europe of thousands of refugees from the turmoil in the Middle East and Africa. This, of course, poses enormous challenges to Europe's existing health care systems.

Europe is currently confronted with several important issues with regard to the provision of proper health care. The most pressing problem is an ever increasing demand for health care due to the aging population and the influx of thousands of refugees.

[a] Department of Otolaryngology–Head and Neck Surgery, Weill Cornell Medicine, 2315 Broadway, New York, NY 10024, USA; [b] Department of Otolaryngology, University of Pittsburgh School of Medicine, 200 Lothrop Street, Pittsburgh, PA 15213, USA; [c] Department of Otorhinolaryngology, Head and Neck Surgery, Paracelsus Medical University, Müllner Hauptstraße 48, Salzburg 5020, Austria
* Corresponding author.
E-mail address: mas9390@med.cornell.edu

Otolaryngol Clin N Am 51 (2018) 675–684
https://doi.org/10.1016/j.otc.2018.01.012
oto.theclinics.com

This problem is compounded by the aging of physicians as a group, many of whom are expected to leave the workforce in the upcoming years. Yet another demographic issue is the increase in the number of women graduating from medical school, many of whom choose to practice either part time or not at all because of family obligations.

The dramatic expansion of the European Union (EU) in 2004 and 2007 increased the pool of physicians overall. However, the countries that were admitted were mostly from Central and Eastern Europe, which are generally thought not to have the same high level of health care as Western Europe. In addition, many physicians from the Middle East and Africa have immigrated to Europe to enjoy the benefits of better career opportunities, increased salaries, and better working and living conditions.

To live up to the motto of the EU, United in Diversity, the medical component of the EU must evolve systems of high-quality medical education across the EU countries. Better organization is necessary for the training of specialists, which is now too lengthy and haphazard. Fellowships in subspecialty areas do not exist as known in the United States.

As important as the foregoing, is the need for an EU-wide system of certifying physicians. Currently, this process is highly developed in some countries and not at all in others. Such a system will be helpful in guarding against physicians who are products of substandard medical education programs being allowed to provide health care in the EU.

GEOPOLITICAL CHANGES FROM THE TWENTIETH TO THE TWENTY-FIRST CENTURY

To understand the nuances of European health care it is important to take into consideration geopolitical events of the twentieth century. After World War II, an initiative was introduced to end wars between the European countries. The European Coal and Steel Community, established by the Treaty of Paris in 1951, and the European Economic Community, established by the Treaty of Rome in 1957, started the economic and political unification of the European countries. The 6 founding European Communities member states were Belgium, France, Western Germany, Italy, Luxembourg, and the Netherlands.[1]

In 1973, Denmark, Ireland, and the United Kingdom joined the European Communities. The removal of General Franco of Spain in 1975 ended dictatorship in Europe. Greece became the tenth member state in 1981, followed by Spain and Portugal in 1986. The Single European Act in 1986 created the Single Market, providing the free flow of trade across borders. The Berlin Wall came down in 1989, opening the border between the East and West Germany, leading to the reunification of Germany in 1990. The rapid collapse of the Soviet Union and communism across Central and Eastern Europe that followed increased communication between Eastern and Western European countries. The Maastricht Treaty, signed in 1992, formally established the EU. In 1993, the Single Market was completed, guaranteeing the 4 freedoms: the free movement of goods, capital, services, and labor within the EU.[1]

In 1990, the Schengen agreement abolished the internal border control and introduced a common visa policy. Elimination of internal borders, increasing use of cell phones, and the Internet allowed easier communication between the European countries. Austria, Finland, and Sweden joined the EU in 1995. On January 1, 1999, the Euro was introduced in 11 countries for commercial and financial transactions only, followed by notes and coins for daily use. The Euro is now the official currency in 19 EU member countries. The Czech Republic, Estonia, Hungary, Latvia, Lithuania, Poland, Slovakia, and Slovenia became members of the EU in 2004, finally ending the political division between East and West. In 2013, Croatia became the 28th member of the EU.[1]

Over the past 2 decades the number of immigrants from outside of EU has increased dramatically. Despite the political controversy on immigration, many European countries rely on migrants to fill work positions, including in the health care sector, owing to labor shortages resulting from continuously falling birth rates and aging of the population.[2] Recent unrest and war in the Middle East and Northern Africa lead to many people fleeing their homes and seeking refuge in various European countries. Germany has been the main destination country for migrants to Europe. In 2015, Germany recorded the highest number of asylum applications compared with previous years, Syria being the main country of origin. The country had 2.14 million registered immigrants for that year, a 46% increase from 2014.[3] The migrants from outside of the EU often face challenges associated with language barrier, integration into a new community, and access to proper health care. However, most of the migrants tend to be young and willing to work, offering a considerable long-term contribution to the European economy.[4]

MEDICAL EDUCATION

After graduation from high school, European students can apply directly to medical schools. Just as the rest of the education in European countries, most of the medical schools are affiliated with state-funded universities and are tuition free. There are an increasing number of government-accredited private universities developing in Europe that require individual tuition fees. It takes 6 years, on average, to complete medical school. Doctorate degrees such as a PhD can be earned during medical school with completion of additional academic work and, in many European countries, successful completion of an academic thesis.

POSTGRADUATE TRAINING

Medical school graduates may apply for residency in a specialty area. The curriculum for each specialty is defined by individual national guidelines and varies in content and duration among different European countries. An otolaryngology residency takes 3 to 6 years, depending on the country. Because there are differences in the curriculum for medical school and residency training among the European countries, transferring between the academic institutions of different countries is not possible without application and approval from the Ministry of Health of that country.

In some European countries, general medical training is required before starting a residency. For example, in the United Kingdom, the 2-year Foundation Programme is recommended.[5] In 2015, Austria introduced an equivalent 1-year general medical training before entering specialty training.

The residency curriculum in otolaryngology varies between the European countries. In general, training is focused on the entire field of otolaryngology without subspecialization. Dedicated subspecialty training during residency is uncommon. In Austria, for example, residents have the option to do an additional 2-year training in laryngology. In the United Kingdom, subspecialty training in the areas of head and neck surgery, otology, skull base surgery, thyroid and parathyroid surgery, rhinology, facial plastic surgery, pediatrics, and laryngology can be a part of the final years of residency training.[6] However, in most EU countries subspecialty training follows residency.

After completing an otolaryngology residency program, the options are to stay in the hospital as an employee with pursuit of subspecialization depending on the opportunities available in the hospital, or to be a general otolaryngologist. The general framework of the office practice depends on the individual country's regulations by the National Ministry of Health and the insurance companies. In Austria, for example, general otolaryngologists in private practice usually do not perform surgery, whereas in Germany surgical practice in the private setting is quite common. Dual affiliation with a hospital and private practice is also available in some countries.

Subspecialty training is done in the hospital setting under mentorship by senior physicians. Pediatric otorhinolaryngology in many European countries is not a defined subspecialty as it is in the United States and children with otolaryngologic disorders are usually treated by the general otolaryngologist. However, after the first gathering of specialists with a focus on pediatric otolaryngology from numerous countries in the 1950s, the European Society of Pediatric Otorhinolaryngology (ESPO) was formed.[7] Independent departments for pediatric otolaryngology are found in the United Kingdom, Poland, Hungary, Italy, Romania, Bulgaria, France, Czech Republic, and Slovak Republic.

Academic medicine has a venerable history in Europe, with the first medical university established in Salerno, Italy, circa 1000 AC.[8] Today, academic work such as medical education and research is usually accomplished in hospitals affiliated with universities. Academic appointments in otolaryngology depend on national and university specific requirements. In German-speaking countries, the academic rank of Doctor Habilitatus describes a lecturer in a specific scientific field; for example, otorhinolaryngology. After employment by a university, the academic title Privatdozent is awarded by the university. A professor title can be achieved subsequently by demonstrating further academic accomplishments, which in turn provides an opportunity to hold a chair position in otolaryngology.

PHYSICIAN COMPETENCY AND CERTIFICATION ACROSS THE EUROPEAN COUNTRIES

Because of the differences in medical education and residency curriculum across the European countries, there is a need for standardized education and certification across Europe. The Association for Medical Education in Europe (AMEE) was founded in 1972 in Copenhagen, Denmark. The goal was to foster communication among medical educators and to help promote national associations for medical education throughout Europe.[9]

In 1984, the American Austrian Foundation (AAF) was established. It is a nonprofit, nongovernmental organization with a goal of fostering exchange in medicine, communications, science, and the arts. The AAF's largest program, the Open Medical Institute (OMI), was established in 1993. It conducts several programs that enable participants, most from Eastern European countries, to learn how medicine is practiced in other countries, and affords them an opportunity for seminars, observerships, and distance learning.[10]

The European Examination Board of Otorhinolaryngology was created by the European Union of Medical Specialists (UEMS) Otorhinolaryngology Section and Board in 2008. The goal was to help standardize the knowledge base among otolaryngologists throughout Europe. Because some European countries have national examinations to evaluate the knowledge acquired during training, the European Board examination is not considered to be an alternative to a national examination.[11]

HEALTH CARE JOB MARKET

Health care is among the most significant sectors of in the EU economy. In 2014, there were approximately 1.8 million practicing physicians in the EU. Germany, Italy, France, the United Kingdom, and Spain have the largest overall number of practicing physicians, and these countries have a combined total of 64% of the practicing physicians in the EU. However, physician density gives a slightly different perspective. Greece has the highest number of physicians per capita, 6.3 physicians per 1000 people, followed by Austria, Portugal, and Lithuania.[12] Poland has the lowest number of physicians per capita in the EU at 2.3 physicians per 1000 people, and the United Kingdom is only slightly higher at 2.8 per 1000. Many of the Balkan countries and the former Soviet republics in Eastern Europe also have low physician density, less than 3.0 per 1000. The number of specialists such as otolaryngologists is even more unevenly distributed among the EU countries (**Table 1**).[13] Among the Western European countries, the United Kingdom has the lowest number of otolaryngologists per capita. It is estimated that 15% of general practitioners workload is otolaryngology-related. Despite the apparent need, NHS financial deficits present a challenge in expanding the number of otolaryngologists.[14]

Between 2004 and 2014, the overall proportion of female physicians has risen from 41% to 48% in the EU. There is a significant difference between the EU countries in regards to the percentage of female physicians. For example, almost 75% of the total number of physicians in Estonia and Latvia are women, in comparison to Luxemburg, Cyprus, Malta, and Belgium, where women make up less than 40% of the total number of physicians.[12]

The demand for health care has been increasing, due to the aging population and immigration. Europe is facing a potential problem with a shortage of physicians, especially in certain geographic locations. According to the European Commission it is estimated that there will be shortage of 230,000 physicians by 2020. There is already an undersupply of physicians in rural areas, and oversupply in the urban areas, particularly in Germany.[12]

Aging of physicians themselves is among the factors affecting the health care sector. In 2012, approximately one-third of all physicians in the EU were 55 year old or older. According to the European Commission's Directorate-General for Health and Food Safety, 3.2% of physicians are expected to leave the workforce by 2020.[15] Another factor affecting the health care market is a more rapid increase in the number of specialists rather than general practitioners.

Physician retention is also an issue facing health care. Despite the requirement of high skill levels and demanding working conditions, the wages tend to be lower than in other professions. Life style has become an important factor influencing physician retention, especially with the increase in the percentage of women medical school graduates. Despite that more 50% of medical students are women, women are still significantly underrepresented in senior academic positions and as department heads.[16] In the United Kingdom only 11% of academic faculty are women, 2 out of 33 are department heads,[17] and 1 in 5 medical schools do not have a female professor.[18] Women career choices and career progression are thought to be mostly affected by family obligations,[19] working part time and taking career breaks.[20]

Member States in the in the EU recognize the professional qualifications of other member states. European physician's certificates are automatically recognized and doctors are allowed to practice anywhere in the EU. This allows many physicians to seek jobs in other EU countries. Expansion of the EU in 2004 and 2007 increased the pool of physicians. Better career opportunities, better salaries, and better working conditions are major factors influencing the movement of physicians between the European states. Physician migration is higher to the Northern and Western EU member states, which leads to uneven distribution and a shortage of certain specialists in some countries. There is also an outflow of physicians to non-EU countries such as Switzerland, the United States, Australia, New Zealand, and Canada. Because of the health care workforce shortage, EU countries rely on recruitment of physicians

Table 1
Distribution of otolaryngologists per country in Europe

Country	Population[a]	Total Number of Otolaryngologists per Country[a]	Number of Otolaryngologists per Population (100,000)[a]	Number of Physicians per Population (100,000)[b]	Percent (%) of Otolaryngologists Among All Physicians
Albania	3,581,655	85	2.4	128.6	1.8
Andorra	71,201	NA	NA	NA	NA
Austria	8,773,700	723	8.2	515.0	1.6
Belarus	10,293,011	90	0.9	407.0	0.2
Belgium	10,379,067	701	6.8	297.1	2.3
Bosnia & Herzegovina	4,498,976	NA	NA	188.6	NA
Bulgaria	7,385,367	130	1.8	399.9	0.4
Croatia	4,494,749	335	7.5	312.6	2.4
Czech Republic	10,235,455	865	8.5	367.7	2.3
Denmark	5,450,661	640	11.7	364.8	3.2
Estonia	1,324,333	104	7.9	331.6	2.4
Faroe Islands	47,246	NA	NA	NA	NA
Finland	5,231,372	491	9.4	300.9	3.1
France	60,876,136	3060	5.0	322.7	1.6
Germany	82,422,299	3312	4.0	412.5	1.0
Gibraltar	27,928	NA	NA	NA	NA
Greece	10,688,058	1400	13.1	625.5	2.1
Guernsey	65,409	NA	NA	NA	NA
Hungary	9,981,334	652	6.5	331.6	2.0
Iceland	299,388	70	23.4	379.1	6.2
Ireland	4,062,235	53	1.3	278.9	0.5
Isle of Man	75,441	NA	NA	NA	NA
Italy	58,133,509	2450	4.2	394.5	1.1
Jersey	91,084	NA	NA	NA	NA
Latvia	2,274,735	150	6.6	322.3	2.0
Liechtenstein	33,987	NA	NA	NA	NA
Lithuania	3,585,906	NA	NA	433.0	NA
Luxembourg	474,413	33	7.0	292.0	2.4
Macedonia	2,050,554	NA	NA	280.0	NA
Malta	400,214	NA	NA	390.8	NA
Moldova	4,466,706	70	1.6	253.7	0.6
Monaco	32,543	NA	NA	NA	NA
Netherlands	16,491,461	548	3.3	335.2	1.0
Norway	4,610,820	340	7.4	442.0	1.7
Poland	38,536,869	1800	4.7	227.1	2.1
Portugal	10,605,870	704	6.6	442.6	1.5
Romania	22,303,552	130	0.6	266.9	0.2

(continued on next page)

Table 1
(continued)

Country	Population[a]	Total Number of Otolaryngologists per Country[a]	Number of Otolaryngologists per Population (100,000)[a]	Number of Physicians per Population (100,000)[b]	Percent (%) of Otolaryngologists Among All Physicians
San Marino	29,251	NA	NA	NA	NA
Serbia	9,396,411	450	4.8	246.3	1.9
Slovakia	5,439,448	476	8.8	338.7	2.6
Slovenia	2,010,347	111	5.5	276.5	2.0
Spain	40,397,842	NA	NA	381.9	NA
Sweden	9,016,596	800	8.9	410.7	2.2
Switzerland	7,523,934	397	5.3	411.4	1.3
Ukraine	**46,710,816**	**210**	**0.4**	**300.0**	**0.1**
United Kingdom	**60,609,153**	**924**	**1.5**	**280.6**	**0.5**

Bolded are the countries with number less than the WHO recommended 2 otolaryngologists per 100,000.

[a] Data from International Federation of Oto-rhino-laryngological Societies database.
[b] Data from WHO database, varying in the years of data acquisition (2007–2015).
Data from European Union. The history of the European Union. Available at: https://europa.eu/european-union/about-eu/history; and Rechel B, Mladovsky P, Ingleby D, et al. Migration and health in an increasingly diverse Europe. Lancet 2013;381(9873):1235–45.

from outside the EU.[21] Because clinical experience and level of training vary tremendously from country to country, establishing a standardized certification program could help assure the uniform and high-quality health care.

HEALTH CARE STRUCTURE AND COVERAGE

The structure of health care systems in Europe differs from country to country. In the EU more than half of the physicians are used by hospitals. For example, in France 82% of physicians are used by hospitals, while in Belgium 23% of physicians are used by the hospitals.[12]

The first social security health care system for workers was established in Germany by Chancellor Otto von Bismarck in 1883.[22] The first National Healthcare System (NHS) was established by the British economist William Henry Beveridge in 1946.[23] The NHS is financed through income tax, controlled by the government, and health care is provided by the government institutions. The social security systems are financed by employer contributions and the government has less influence on these systems.

Current health care systems in individual countries throughout Europe are complex and are constantly undergoing changes and revisions. However, 3 basic types of health care structures are found across Europe. One structure is government-provided insurance and provision of care through a public health service such as the NHS in the United Kingdom and similar systems in Italy, Spain, and Sweden. The second model is a government-funded and government-regulated insurance such as the Social Security System in France, with most doctors working in private settings. A third model is government-regulated but privately managed insurance companies and provision of care. The latter is found in Switzerland and the Netherlands. Regardless of the model, private insurance is often available in most

European health care systems, usually as a voluntary addition to the basic government insurance plan.

Depending on the health care system, physician reimbursement is usually provided by either government or insurance companies. National formulas for reimbursement are rather complex and are influenced by the government, economic factors, and private institutions. In Germany and Austria, physicians negotiate contracts and reimbursement directly with the insurance companies.

In 2006, the German Social Security System spent 10.6% of its gross domestic product on health care.[24] However, in Germany, dissatisfaction with health care is rising for reasons that are unclear. In 2002, a survey performed by the Fritz Beske Institut für Gesundheits-System-Forschung revealed that 42% of people when asked whether the health care system in Germany provides high-quality care answered "somewhat no" or "no."[24] One possible explanation might be the growing complexity of a system overwhelmed by demographic and economic changes.

Even though each national health care system is organized and financed through its own country, there are EU policies aimed to provide the best possible health care for all European member states by financial, structural, and informational support. In 2007, the EU adopted a health strategy based on 4 principles: (1) European shared health values, (2) health is the greatest wealth, (3) consideration about health must be included in all policies, and (4) the EU voice must be heard on all issues affecting global health. Three main objectives of European health care are to improve health in an aging population, protect the European citizens from health threats, and to support dynamic health systems and new technologies.[25]

Any European citizen has a right to health care even outside of the EU. European insurance plans provide reimbursement of payment for health care received in non-EU countries. It is the patient's responsibility to file for a reimbursement from the insurance company after receiving treatment outside the system. The amount of reimbursement depends on the individual's insurance contract.[26]

For health care coverage, more expensive private insurance plans allow for more flexibility and options for access to health care providers. However, in Europe, each citizen is required by law to have health insurance. The idea is that everyone has to have access to basic health care, even in case of unemployment.

SUMMARY

Europe is among the most populated geographic regions of the world with a complex geopolitical history and culturally diverse population. EU, as it exists today, stands for a modern international community of wealth and growth, with political, economic, and sociologic developments based on the principles of diplomacy and exchange between member states and the world. However, health care systems are still mainly managed and organized on a national level. The objective of the EU programs is to establish sustainable health care systems that address health care workforce shortages while facilitating innovative and quality health care. It is also essential to establish standardized medical training and certification to address concerns of uneven quality of health care, as well as workforce shortages, across the European countries.

REFERENCES

1. Official website of the European Union. History. Available at: https://europa.eu/european-union/about-eu/history. Accessed October 22, 2017.
2. Rechel B, Mladovsky P, Ingleby D, et al. Migration and health in an increasingly diverse Europe. Lancet 2013;381(9873):1235–45.

3. Migration report 2015–central conclusions. Federal Office for Migration and Refugees (BAMF). Available at: http://www.polen.diplo.de/contentblob/4450184/Daten/7213830/migrationsbericht2015.pdf. Accessed October 22, 2017.

4. Permanand G, Krasnik A, Kluge H, et al. Europe's migration challenges: mounting an effective health system response. Eur J Public Health 2016;26(1):3–4.

5. General medical council. Available at: www.gmc-uk.org. Accessed October 22, 2017.

6. SFOUK. ENT training structure. Available at: http://sfo.entuk.org/training-structure. Accessed October 22, 2017.

7. Official website of the European Society of Pediatric Otorhinolaryngology. Available at: http://www.espo.eu.com/brief-history/. Accessed October 22, 2017.

8. Fisch S. Geschichte Der Europäischen Universität. München: ©Verlag C.H.Beck oHG; 2015.

9. AMEE Association for Medical Education in Europe. Available at: https://amee.org/what-is-amee. Accessed October 22, 2017.

10. The American Austrian Foundation. Available at: http://aaf-online.org/. Accessed October 22, 2017.

11. European Board Examination in Otorhinolaryngology–Head and Neck Surgery by the UEMS–ORL section. Available at: http://www.ebeorl-hns.org/. Accessed October 22, 2017.

12. Eurostat statistic explained. Health in the European Union–facts and figures. Available at: http://ec.europa.eu/eurostat/statistics-explained. Accessed October 22, 2017.

13. World Health Organization. Global health observatory (GHO) data. Available at: http://www.who.int/gho/health_workforce/physicians_density/en/.   Accessed October 22, 2017.

14. Powell S. So you want to be an ENT surgeon. London: BMJ Careers; 2007. Availabe at: http://careers.bmj.com/careers/advice/view-article.html?id=2391. Accessed October 22, 2017.

15. The European Commission's Directorate-General Health and Food Safety. Available at: http://ec.europa.eu/dgs/health_food-safety/index_en.htm. Accessed October 22, 2017.

16. British Medical Association. Women in academic medicine. Developing equality in governance and management for career progression. London: BMA; 2008. Available at: http://www.bma.org.uk/images/Womenacademicmedicine_tcm41-178228.pdf. Accessed October 22, 2017.

17. Medical Schools Council. Women in clinical academia. Attracting and developing the Medical and Dental Workforce of the Future. London: Medical Schools Council; 2007.

18. Sandhu B, Margerison C, Holdcroft A. Women in the UK medical academic workforce. Med Educ 2007;41:909–14.

19. Allen I. Women doctors and their careers what now? BMJ 2005;331:569–72.

20. Taylor KS, Lambert TW, Goldacre MJ. Career progression and destinations, comparing men and women in the NHS: postal questionnaire surveys. BMJ 2009;338:b1735.

21. Wismar M, Maier CB, Glinos IA, et al. Health professional mobility and healthcare systems. Evidence from 17 European countries, observatory study series No. 23. Copenhagen (Denmark): European Observatory on Health Systems and Policies, WHO Regional Office for Europe; 2011.

22. Social security history: Otto von Bismarck. Available at: https://www.ssa.gov/history/ottob.html. Accessed October 22, 2017.

23. Gesundheitswesen im Europäischen Vergleich–Ein Überblick. Available at: http://www.bpb.de/politik/innenpolitik/gesundheitspolitik/72906/gesundheitswesen-im-europaeischen-vergleich. Accessed October 22, 2017.

24. Das Gesundheitswesen in Deutschland–Ein Überblick. Available at: http://www.bpb.de/politik/innenpolitik/gesundheitspolitik/72547/gesundheitswesen-im-ueberblick. Accessed October 22, 2017.

25. European Commission. The European Union explained: public health. 2014. Available at: https://ec.europa.eu/health//sites/health/files/health_policies/docs/improving_health_for_all_eu_citizens_en.pdf. Accessed October 22, 2017.

26. Your Europe: health. Available at: http://europa.eu/youreurope/citizens/health/when-living-abroad/healthcare/index_en.htm. Accessed October 22, 2017.

Otolaryngology-Related Disorders in Underserved Populations, Otolaryngology Training and Workforce Considerations in North America

Brian D. Westerberg, MD, MHSc, FRCSC[a], Miriam N. Lango, MD[b,c],*

KEYWORDS

• Disparities • Underserved populations • Otolaryngology workforce • North America

KEY POINTS

• Underserved and vulnerable populations are less frequently diagnosed with common otolaryngologic disorders, yet come to clinical attention with advanced forms of the disorder, suggesting decreased engagement with the health care system.

• Furthermore, limited access to high-quality health care, and socioeconomic, cultural, and biologic risk factors may also contribute to observed differences in care.

• The tendency of vulnerable populations to obtain care by low-volume providers and facilities likely contributes to worse outcomes, and higher health care costs.

• In Canada, greater standardization in care delivery has been achieved by managing head and neck squamous cell cancers at designated regional centers.

• The geographic distribution of providers and facilities suitable to care for complex otolaryngology-related disorders should be optimized to enhance the appropriate and timely delivery of otolaryngology care.

BACKGROUND

Underserved populations within Canada and the United States exhibit poorer health outcomes despite greater per capita health expenditures.[1–3] Disparities in care and health outcomes are regularly observed. These discrepancies are most prominent in

Disclosure Statement: The authors have nothing to disclose.
[a] Division of Otolaryngology–Head and Neck Surgery, Department of Surgery, B.C. Rotary Hearing and Balance Centre, Branch for International Surgical Care, University of British Columbia, 1081 Burrard Street, Providence 2, Vancouver, British Columbia V6Z 1Y6, Canada; [b] Department of Surgical Oncology, Head and Neck Surgery Section, Fox Chase Cancer Center, Temple University Health System, 333 Cottman Avenue, Philadelphia, PA 19111, USA; [c] Department of Otolaryngology, Temple University School of Medicine, 3401 N Broad Street, Philadelphia, PA 19140, USA
* Corresponding author. 333 Cottman Avenue, Philadelphia, PA 19111.
E-mail address: Miriam.Lango@fccc.edu

Otolaryngol Clin N Am 51 (2018) 685–695
https://doi.org/10.1016/j.otc.2018.01.013
0030-6665/18/© 2018 Elsevier Inc. All rights reserved.

oto.theclinics.com

rural and/or remote communities in Canada largely represented by indigenous populations, a diverse group of peoples, including First Nations, Inuit, and Metis, each consisting of hundreds of distinct groups with different language, cultures, history, and geography. In contrast, in the United States, the nature and degree of insurance coverage varies widely, and the underserved population is more heterogeneous, encompassing a variety of socioeconomic, racial, ethnic, and/or rural groups that exhibit less engagement with the health care system. Indigenous populations in the United States are only one of many underserved groups.

UNDERSERVED POPULATIONS

Despite the Canadian Health Care Act, legislation that called for the same level of health care for all Canadian residents, some populations exhibit poorer health. For instance, the life expectancy of First Nations peoples is 5 to 7 years less than the Canadian population's life expectancies, with higher rates of deaths caused by circulatory diseases and injury, higher rates of suicide (five to seven times higher in Aboriginal youths than the national average and 20 times higher in Inuit males), and higher rates of infectious diseases including pertussis (2.2 times higher), rubella (seven times higher), tuberculosis (six times higher), and shigellosis (2.1 times higher).[4]

Approximately 18% (6.5 million people) of Canada's population is considered rural and about 1.1% (400,000 people) is living in remote communities lacking access by road, rail, or water. Of these, approximately 340,000 are indigenous (Statistics Canada, 2015). In the United States, according to the US census, a similar proportion (19.3%) of the population (about 60 million people) reside in rural regions that cover 97% of the land area of the United States.

In the United States, the Health Resources and Services Administration designates both geographic regions and specific populations as medically underserved. Medically underserved areas have shortages of primary care health services within geographic regions, whereas medically underserved populations face economic, cultural, or linguistic barriers to health care engagement. The specificity of such definitions enables the targeting of local, state, and federal resources to specific geographic areas. Under this designation, African Americans and Hispanics are not considered underserved, despite the substantially worse health outcomes for many conditions observed in these groups.

Otolaryngology-related disorders are reviewed here not only in underserved but also vulnerable populations, those groups whose demographic, geographic, or economic characteristics impede or prevent group members' access to health care services.[5] These include the poor, the mentally ill, and those living in remote, rural areas, racial and ethnic minorities, and any social group with disproportionately high rates of adverse health outcomes.[6]

ACCESSIBILITY

A multitude of social determinants of health[7] impact on health care status in vulnerable populations, including race and ethnicity, socioeconomic status, racism and discrimination, historical conditions and colonialism. Underserved and vulnerable populations also exhibit diminished engagement with the health care system, and consequently come to clinical attention less frequently but with advanced disorders.

Health insurance is a prerequisite for timely and effective care but insurance coverage by itself does not guarantee access that leads to timely diagnosis or effective treatment. In the United States, specific health systems and networks were devised to improve access to health care for specific populations, such as the Veterans Affairs and

Indian Health Service. The provision of health care to Indigenous populations in Canada is affected by complicated historical agreements between federal, provincial, municipal, and Indigenous governments that vary across the country.[8] Gaps and ambiguities have created unforeseen barriers to access to care. Rooted in these inequities are also probably, to an equal extent, the distrust inherent in the relationship between Indigenous societies and those of European descent, effects of colonialism on any population, and the loss of "an indigenous consciousness."[9] Arguably, the simple act of forced settlement of indigenous populations contributed significantly to the poor health of their peoples, which may partly explain why large amounts of money spent on government programs have had such limited effect on their health status.

RATES OF DIAGNOSIS AND ENGAGEMENT WITH THE HEALTH CARE SYSTEM

Underserved populations exhibit decreased engagement with the health care system, which is reflected in lower rates of diagnosis but greater disease severity of some common otolaryngology-related disorders.

- Black and Hispanic children are less often diagnosed with frequent ear infections, hay fever, strep pharyngitis, and sinusitis than white children. This is not apparently related to the incidence of these conditions in children but rather reflects lower rates of diagnosis.[10]
- The subtype and severity of chronic sinusitis in adults also varies by race and socioeconomic status. White adults from high-income areas are more likely to be diagnosed with chronic sinusitis of lesser apparent disease severity.[11]
- Similar patterns are observed for malignancies of the head and neck. The incidence of thyroid cancer is lower in regions with greater poverty, percent nonwhite race/ethnicity, and uninsured population, markers of decreased access to health care[12,13]; however, patients with thyroid cancer from such areas present with more advanced stage at initial presentation[12] and are at higher risk of death.[14]
- Race/ethnicity has not only been associated with increased risk of death from well-differentiated thyroid carcinoma,[15] but also advanced larynx cancer,[16,17] and sinonasal carcinoma.[18] Nonwhite patients with head and neck cancer present with greater local tumor burden before treatment, and had worse disease control and survival.[19]
- Associations between insurance status (no insurance or Medicaid insurance) and poor head and neck cancer outcomes have been amply documented in the literature.[20–22] Poor outcomes seem to be a result of the greater prevalence of advanced disease at initial presentation.[23] The causal role of limited access because of health insurance status was supported in a recent study of patients with breast cancer. Disenrollment of 170,000 Tennessee Medicaid enrollees in 2005 was associated with a subsequent 3.3% increase in advanced-stage presentation of breast cancer, and delays in initiating surgery and treatment of women from low-income regions, suggesting that lack of health insurance itself has a substantial negative impact on health outcomes.[24]
- Nevertheless, health insurance coverage does not necessarily guarantee engagement. Patients from lower socioeconomic strata are less compliant with follow-up and surveillance recommendations. Children with Medicaid who undergo unilateral cochlear implantation miss postoperative follow-up visits and develop postoperative complications more frequently than comparable children with private insurance, and less often undergo sequential bilateral cochlear implantation.[25]

BEHAVIORAL RISK FACTORS

- Behaviors that can strongly influence health include tobacco and/or ethanol use, physical activity, nutrition, sexual practices, and screening behaviors. Poverty, remote/rural geography, and nonwhite race/ethnicity are factors associated with increase prevalence of behaviors that produce worse health.
- The development of many head and neck cancers is associated with tobacco and ethanol abuse, behaviors linked with less education, greater poverty, and nonwhite race.[26,27] Tobacco cessation efforts have resulted in a decline in the incidence of tobacco-related malignancies over the last 25 years. Racial disparities in the prevalence of preventable risk factors for head and neck cancer nevertheless persist and may respond to targeted education and prevention programs.[28]
- Intergenerational, historical trauma may account for the adoption of some negative behaviors and reluctance on the part of some groups to engage with the health care system. Children of parents who attended Indian Residential Schools in Canada are more likely to smoke and abuse alcohol.[29] In the United States, the legacy of slavery and abuse including the infamous Tuskegee Syphilis Study is believed to underlie the mistrust of the health care system by African Americans. Such mistrust may prevent patients from obtaining needed care and adhering to recommended life-saving treatments.[30]

HOST AND DISEASE BIOLOGY

Some populations may be intrinsically more susceptible to certain disorders.

- The higher incidence of otitis media in the indigenous populations in North America, particularly in Canada, has been quoted in the literature for decades.[31] Reasons for this to date are speculative but may include genetic, environmental (eg, breast feeding or dietary changes away from traditional high-protein/high-fat diets), access to care, or other socioeconomic factors. Otitis media is an excellent example of the interplay between multiple cofactors and increasing prevalence of a disease in low-resource settings.
- The role of host and biologic factors on head and neck cancer–related outcomes remains controversial. Disparities in outcomes attributable to biologic differences of cancers in African Americans and Hispanics may be exaggerated. In a cohort of 200 patients with head and neck cancer treated at a Veterans Affairs facility, no differences in initial stage, tumor subsite, treatment, guidelines compliant care, and survival between white and black patients were observed.[32] This study evaluated a homogeneous population of veterans from one region, and may be limited by sample size and generalizability, but raises the possibility that patients could expect similar survivals regardless of race or ethnicity if provided with similar access to evidence-based head and neck cancer care.
- The risk factor profile for patients with human papilloma virus (HPV)-associated oropharynx cancers contrasts with that of other head and neck cancers[33] with higher incidence rates among white males.[34] The better survival of patients with HPV-related oropharynx cancer is principally related to less aggressive tumor biology of these cancers, rather than access to care.[35–37] The decreased frequency of HPV-mediated cancer in nonwhite groups largely accounts for differences in disease-specific survival.[38–40] Males and non-Hispanic blacks exhibit less knowledge and awareness of HPV and the HPV vaccine than other groups,[41] suggesting prevention through education could be effective.

LOW-VOLUME PROVIDERS/FACILITIES AND THE FREQUENCY OF INAPPROPRIATE CARE

Vulnerable populations are more likely to receive care that does not conform to evidence-based guidelines by low-volume providers. Nonwhite, Medicaid, or uninsured patients disproportionately undergo major operative procedures at low-volume hospitals.[42] Numerous quality issues including unsupported variation in the use of medical services and procedures have been identified[43,44]:

- Medicaid and nonwhite patients were more likely to undergo pituitary surgery at facilities with lower case volumes, and were more likely to develop postoperative complications.[45]
- Patients from poor communities, who were more likely to undergo thyroidectomy for thyroid cancer than those from wealthier communities, were less likely to undergo surgery by high-volume surgeons.[46,47]

The care obtained by vulnerable populations more frequently violates best evidence-based guidelines recommendations.

- Not only are African American patients more likely to undergo thyroid cancer surgery by low-volume surgeons, they are less likely than white patients to undergo appropriate surgery and adjuvant radioiodine for differentiated thyroid cancer.[48]
- Compared with white patients, African American patients with larynx cancer more often undergo total laryngectomy for T1-3 cancers, and more often undergo primary radiotherapy for T4 larynx cancers.[49] Thus, cancers eligible for organ preservation are treated with laryngectomy; cancers most likely to require laryngectomy for local control and organ dysfunction are treated nonoperatively.

Delays in the initiation of treatment after diagnosis are greater for some populations.

- After diagnosis, the time interval to head and neck cancer treatment initiation significantly varies by race, ethnicity, insurance status, and distance from a treating facility.[50] Delays in initiating treatment of greater than 46 days affects survival, independent of all other factors including tumor stage, suggesting that time to treatment initiation could be used as a quality indicator for institutions treating head and neck cancer.[51]

GEOGRAPHIC VARIATIONS

In the United States, poverty maps to specific geographic regions, and individuals living in those areas engage with local, often underresourced health care facilities. County health rankings assigned by the University of Wisconsin Population Health Institute for every county in the United States, based on a variety of community health indicators, may be used for local needs assessments and program planning.[52] Such health rankings have been largely validated in the otolaryngology literature. Individuals from specific geographic regions have high rates of advanced allergic fungal sinusitis,[53] and poor thyroid surgery outcomes.[46]

Disparities in outcomes based on geographic and regional socioeconomic factors have also been reported in Canada.

- Unwarranted variations in head and neck cancer treatment decrease when managed at Canadian regional centers; the treatment for salivary gland malignancies not managed at regional centers, varies greatly across geographic regions in Canada.[54] Despite regionalization of head and neck cancer treatment to designated high- volume centers, the disease-free and overall survival rates of patients with oral cancer residing in rural Canadian communities is diminished relative to those in urban and intermediate communities.[55]

- Indigenous populations in Canada remain at particularly high risk of poor head and neck cancer outcomes. Oral cavity and pharynx cancer showed an excess mortality rate ratio of 1.54 (95% confidence interval, 1.10–2.18) in First Nations peoples relative to non-Aboriginals.[56] First Nations peoples had poorer survival for nearly all cancers with the exception of multiple myeloma, and income and rurality explained little of these disparities. What is not clear is if this is a consequence of differences in tumor, patient, or health care system factors.

WORKFORCE CONSIDERATIONS

In North America, the supply of physicians varies greatly across geographic regions with relative shortages in some rural areas.[57,58] Even in areas in the United States with many physicians, some physicians restrict or deny new patient visits for patients with unfavorable insurance coverage or Medicaid. Indeed, physicians are less likely to treat patients with unfavorable insurance coverage if they practice in physician-dense areas. States with the lowest percentages of physicians accepting Medicaid include New Jersey (38.7% of physicians), California (54.2%), Florida (55.9%), Louisiana (56.8%), and New York (57.1%). In contrast, 96.5% of physicians in Nebraska accepted new Medicaid patients.[59] Thus, the regions with the highest supplies of physicians also have the greatest proportions of physicians refusing care to Medicaid patients. Otolaryngologists, like other physicians, tend to cluster in physician-dense areas. Physician-population ratios may not accurately reflect otolaryngologists willing to care for underserved or vulnerable populations[60] precluding effective workforce planning.

In Canada, most otolaryngologists/head and neck surgeons (OHNS) practice in urban centers, with a comparative increase in numbers of practicing surgeons over the years 2002 to 2013 in urban centers and a relative decrease practicing in rural settings.[58] An estimate of provision of otolaryngologic care to indigenous communities showed only 4.9% of population centers with Indigenous peoples had an OHNS provider with the remaining 94.7% population centers with Indigenous peoples having no OHNS providers. OHNS care is often provided to rural and remote areas in Canada via telemedicine or seasonal visits.

The regionalization of complex surgeries has increased over time in Canada and the United States, probably as a combined consequence of attempting to maintain high volumes and better outcomes in centralized locations and partly perhaps because new graduates choose to perform less variety of surgical procedures. In the United States, despite an absence of central planning, complex head and neck surgery is nevertheless increasingly conducted in regional hubs.[61] As a result of changes in practice patterns, some have called for changes in the nature and goals of otolaryngology training in the United States.[62] The need for otolaryngologists to offer comprehensive surgical services has declined. Complex otolaryngology-related surgeries may be directed to a smaller number of well-trained, high-volume surgeons.

THE ROLE OF HEALTH CARE ORGANIZATIONS IN DISPARITIES IN CARE AND OUTCOME

Vulnerable populations frequently obtain care at safety-net hospitals (those that provide care for low-income, exploitable, or uninsured populations). The reported surgical outcomes of patients treated at safety net hospitals are generally less favorable. Yet, head and neck cancer surgery at safety net hospitals has not been associated with higher rates of hospital-acquired conditions.[63,64] Of uninsured and Medicaid patients with larynx cancer, those treated at academic and teaching hospitals have better short- and long-term survival than those treated at other types of facilities.[65] The high degree of regionalization for head and neck cancer surgery could be contributing to these favorable trends. Nevertheless, some of the neediest and sickest patients with head and neck cancer who could benefit from care at tertiary care centers continue to obtain head and neck cancer care at low-volume community hospitals.[66]

GEOGRAPHIC DISTRIBUTION OF RESIDENCY TRAINING PROGRAMS IN THE UNITED STATES

Otolaryngology residency training programs have been established in geographic areas with the greatest population densities. Regions with the greatest number of otolaryngology residency programs also have the largest per capita concentrations of otolaryngologists (without including trainees), and such areas spend more on otolaryngology physician services.[67] When designated federal funds for residency training are included, regional spending is even greater. Hence, rural and remote populations, regardless of ethnicity or cultural background, are underserved as a result. This has prompted calls for establishing rural-based surgical training programs.[68–70]

In many areas, a limited number of institutions and providers absorb the cost of caring for the uninsured and underinsured, receiving additional payment for managing vulnerable populations. Such hospitals benefitted most from Medicaid expansion under the Affordable Care Act.[71] Even if the Affordable Care Act is not repealed and replaced, disproportionate share payments to hospitals for uncompensated care will be reduced starting in 2018, in states with and without Medicaid expansion. The number of acute care hospitals has decreased over the last 30 years, unable to survival economically in an increasingly competitive health care environment. A greater proportion of closures occurred among public hospitals. Consequently, the care of the indigent has increasingly been shifted to the private sector.[72] Such trends are likely to continue, and will likely make it increasingly difficult to meet the health care needs of poor and uninsured populations.

SUMMARY

Health disparities are caused by complex, multidirectional interactions that link biologic, clinical, organizational, and broader social influences. Although biologic processes play a role in the clinical phenotype of some otolaryngology disorders, health care access and health system organizational factors unquestionably contribute to the disparate health outcomes observed in some populations. Although health disparities have been amply documented in otolaryngology and the broader medical literature, the best means by which to diminish disparities in care is not entirely clear. Cross-sectional studies may exhibit differences in treatments and outcomes, but do not always suggest simple and effective solutions. The current health systems in North American face substantial challenges. Accurate data are needed to improve accountability and eventually enhance outcomes.

REFERENCES

1. Young TK, Chatwood S. Health care in the North: what Canada can learn from its circumpolar neighbours. Can Med Assoc J 2011;183(2):209–14.

2. Oosterveer TM, Young TK. Primary health care accessibility challenges in remote indigenous communities in Canada's north. Int J Circumpolar Health 2015;74: 29576.
3. Waters H, Steinhardt L, Oliver TR, et al. The costs of non-insurance in Maryland. J Health Care Poor Underserved 2007;18(1):139–51.
4. Canada IPAo, Canada TAoFoMo. First Nations, Inuit, Métis Health CORE COMPE-TENCIES: a curriculum framework for undergraduate medical education. 2009. Available at: https://afmc.ca/pdf/CoreCompetenciesEng.pdf. Accessed February 17, 2018.
5. Gruca TS, Nam I, Tracy R. Reaching rural patients through otolaryngology visiting consultant clinics. Otolaryngol Head Neck Surg 2014;151(6):895–8.
6. Flaskerud JH, Winslow BJ. Conceptualizing vulnerable populations health-related research. Nurs Res 1998;47(2):69–78.
7. Reading JL, Gideon V, Kmetic AM, et al. First Nations wholistic policy and planning model: discussion paper for the World Health Organization Commission on social determinants of health. Ottawa, Ontario: Assembly of First Nations; 2007.
8. National Collaborating Centre for Aboriginal Health. An overview of Aboriginal health in Canada. British Columbia, Canada: NCCAH; 2013.
9. Alfred GT. Colonialism and state dependency. J Aborig Health 2009;5(2):42–60.
10. Shay S, Shapiro NL, Bhattacharyya N. Pediatric otolaryngologic conditions: racial and socioeconomic disparities in the United States. Laryngoscope 2017;127(3): 746–52.
11. Lu-Myers Y, Deal AM, Miller JD, et al. Comparison of socioeconomic and demographic factors in patients with chronic rhinosinusitis and allergic fungal rhinosinusitis. Otolaryngol Head Neck Surg 2015;153(1):137–43.
12. Morris LG, Sikora AG, Myssiorek D, et al. The basis of racial differences in the incidence of thyroid cancer. Ann Surg Oncol 2008;15(4):1169–76.
13. Morris LG, Sikora AG, Tosteson TD, et al. The increasing incidence of thyroid cancer: the influence of access to care. Thyroid 2013;23(7):885–91.
14. Harari A, Li N, Yeh MW. Racial and socioeconomic disparities in presentation and outcomes of well-differentiated thyroid cancer. J Clin Endocrinol Metab 2014; 99(1):133–41.
15. Krook KA, Fedewa SA, Chen AY. Prognostic indicators in well-differentiated thyroid carcinoma when controlling for stage and treatment. Laryngoscope 2015;125(4):1021–7.
16. Chen AY, Fedewa S, Zhu J. Temporal trends in the treatment of early- and advanced-stage laryngeal cancer in the United States, 1985-2007. Arch Otolaryngol Head Neck Surg 2011;137(10):1017–24.
17. Chen AY, Halpern M. Factors predictive of survival in advanced laryngeal cancer. Arch Otolaryngol Head Neck Surg 2007;133(12):1270–6.
18. Patel ZM, Li J, Chen AY, et al. Determinants of racial differences in survival for sinonasal cancer. Laryngoscope 2016;126(9):2022–8.
19. Qureshi MM, Romesser PB, Ajani A, et al. Race disparities attributed to volumetric tumor burden in patients with head and neck cancer treated with radiotherapy. Head Neck 2016;38(1):126–34.
20. Walker GV, Grant SR, Guadagnolo BA, et al. Disparities in stage at diagnosis, treatment, and survival in nonelderly adult patients with cancer according to insurance status. J Clin Oncol 2014;32(28):3118–25.
21. Chen AY, Schrag NM, Halpern M, et al. Health insurance and stage at diagnosis of laryngeal cancer: does insurance type predict stage at diagnosis? Arch Otolaryngol Head Neck Surg 2007;133(8):784–90.

22. Kwok J, Langevin SM, Argiris A, et al. The impact of health insurance status on the survival of patients with head and neck cancer. Cancer 2010;116(2):476–85.
23. Subramanian S, Chen A. Treatment patterns and survival among low-income Medicaid patients with head and neck cancer. JAMA Otolaryngol Head Neck Surg 2013;139(5):489–95.
24. Tarazi WW, Bradley CJ, Bear HD, et al. Impact of Medicaid disenrollment in Tennessee on breast cancer stage at diagnosis and treatment. Cancer 2017;123(17): 3312–9.
25. Chang DT, Ko AB, Murray GS, et al. Lack of financial barriers to pediatric cochlear implantation: impact of socioeconomic status on access and outcomes. Arch Otolaryngol Head Neck Surg 2010;136(7):648–57.
26. Sturgis EM, Cinciripini PM. Trends in head and neck cancer incidence in relation to smoking prevalence: an emerging epidemic of human papillomavirus-associated cancers? Cancer 2007;110(7):1429–35.
27. Rohlfing ML, Mays AC, Isom S, et al. Insurance status as a predictor of mortality in patients undergoing head and neck cancer surgery. Laryngoscope 2017; 127(12):2784–9.
28. Dwojak S, Bhattacharyya N. Racial disparities in preventable risk factors for head and neck cancer. Laryngoscope 2017;127(5):1068–72.
29. Bombay A, Matheson K, Anisman H. The intergenerational effects of Indian Residential Schools: implications for the concept of historical trauma. Transcult Psychiatry 2014;51(3):320–38.
30. Gaston GB, Alleyne-Green B. The impact of African Americans' beliefs about HIV medical care on treatment adherence: a systematic review and recommendations for interventions. AIDS Behav 2013;17(1):31–40.
31. Bowd AD. Otitis media: health and social consequences for aboriginal youth in Canada's north. Int J Circumpolar Health 2005;64(1):5–15.
32. Sandulache VC, Kubik MW, Skinner HD, et al. Impact of race/ethnicity on laryngeal cancer in patients treated at a Veterans Affairs Medical Center. Laryngoscope 2013;123(9):2170–5.
33. Gillison ML, D'Souza G, Westra W, et al. Distinct risk factor profiles for human papillomavirus type 16-positive and human papillomavirus type 16-negative head and neck cancers. J Natl Cancer Inst 2008;100(6):407–20.
34. Chaturvedi AK, Engels EA, Anderson WF, et al. Incidence trends for human papillomavirus–related and –unrelated oral squamous cell carcinomas in the United States. J Clin Oncol 2008;26(4):612–9.
35. Mellin H, Friesland S, Lewensohn R, et al. Human papillomavirus (HPV) DNA in tonsillar cancer: clinical correlates, risk of relapse, and survival. Int J Cancer 2000;89(3):300–4.
36. Gillison ML, Koch WM, Capone RB, et al. Evidence for a causal association between human papillomavirus and a subset of head and neck cancers. J Natl Cancer Inst 2000;92(9):709–20.
37. Mork J, Lie AK, Glattre E, et al. Human papillomavirus infection as a risk factor for squamous-cell carcinoma of the head and neck. N Engl J Med 2001;344(15): 1125–31.
38. Jiron J, Sethi S, Ali-Fehmi R, et al. Racial disparities in human papillomavirus (HPV) associated head and neck cancer. Am J Otolaryngol 2014;35(2):147–53.
39. Schrank TP, Han Y, Weiss H, et al. Case-matching analysis of head and neck squamous cell carcinoma in racial and ethnic minorities in the United States: possible role for human papillomavirus in survival disparities. Head Neck 2011; 33(1):45–53.

40. Ragin C, Liu JC, Jones G, et al. Prevalence of HPV infection in racial-ethnic sub-groups of head and neck cancer patients. Carcinogenesis 2016 [Epub ahead of print].

41. Boakye EA, Tobo BB, Osazuwa-Peters N. Abstract A51: racial and gender disparities in knowledge and awareness of HPV and HPV vaccine in a national sample of U.S. adults. Cancer Epidemiol Biomarkers Prev 2016;25(3 Suppl):A51.

42. Liu JH, Zingmond DS, McGory ML, et al. Disparities in the utilization of high-volume hospitals for complex surgery. JAMA 2006;296(16):1973–80.

43. Smedley BD, Stith AY, Nelson AR. Unequal treatment: confronting racial and ethnic disparities in health care. Washington, DC: National Academies Press (US); 2003. Available at: https://www.ncbi.nlm.nih.gov/books/NBK220358/. Accessed February 17, 2018.

44. MacKenzie AR, Parker I. Introduction to quality issues in vulnerable populations. J Oncol Pract 2015;11(3):185–6.

45. Goljo E, Parasher AK, Iloreta AM, et al. Racial, ethnic, and socioeconomic disparities in pituitary surgery outcomes. Laryngoscope 2016;126(4):808–14.

46. Al-Qurayshi Z, Randolph GW, Srivastav S, et al. Outcomes in thyroid surgery are affected by racial, economic, and healthcare system demographics. Laryngoscope 2016;126(9):2194–9.

47. Al-Qurayshi Z, Randolph GW, Srivastav S, et al. Outcomes in endocrine cancer surgery are affected by racial, economic, and healthcare system demographics. Laryngoscope 2016;126(3):775–81.

48. Shah SA, Adam MA, Thomas SM, et al. Racial disparities in differentiated thyroid cancer: have we bridged the gap? Thyroid 2017;27(6):762–72.

49. Shin JY, Truong MT. Racial disparities in laryngeal cancer treatment and outcome: a population-based analysis of 24,069 patients. Laryngoscope 2015;125(7):1667–74.

50. Murphy CT, Galloway TJ, Handorf EA, et al. Increasing time to treatment initiation for head and neck cancer: an analysis of the National Cancer Database. Cancer 2015;121(8):1204–13.

51. Murphy CT, Galloway TJ, Handorf EA, et al. Survival impact of increasing time to treatment initiation for patients with head and neck cancer in the United States. J Clin Oncol 2015;34(2):169–78.

52. Peppard PE, Kindig DA, Dranger E, et al. Ranking community health status to stimulate discussion of local public health issues: the Wisconsin County health rankings. Am J Public Health 2008;98(2):209–12.

53. Miller JD, Deal AM, McKinney KA, et al. Markers of disease severity and socio-economic factors in allergic fungal rhinosinusitis. Int Forum Allergy Rhinol 2014;4(4):272–9.

54. Eskander A, Irish J, Freeman J, et al. Overview of major salivary gland cancer surgery in Ontario (2003-2010). J Otolaryngol Head Neck Surg 2014;43:50.

55. Zhang H, Dziegielewski PT, Nguyen TT, et al. The effects of geography on survival in patients with oral cavity squamous cell carcinoma. Oral Oncol 2015;51(6):578–85.

56. Withrow DR, Pole JD, Nishri ED, et al. Cancer survival disparities between first nation and non-aboriginal adults in Canada: follow-up of the 1991 census mortality cohort. Cancer Epidemiol Biomarkers Prev 2017;26(1):145–51.

57. Cooper RA. Seeking a balanced physician workforce for the 21st century. JAMA 1994;272(9):680–7.

58. Crowson M, Lin V. The Canadian otolaryngology-HNS workforce in the urban-rural continuum: longitudinal data from 2002-2013. Otolaryngol Head Neck Surg 2018; 158(1):127–34.

59. Hing E, Decker S, Jamoom E. Acceptance of new patients with public and private insurance by office-based physicians: United States, 2013. NCHS Data Brief 2015;(195):1–8.

60. Lango MN, Handorf E, Arjmand E. The geographic distribution of the otolaryngology workforce in the United States. Laryngoscope 2017;127(1):95–101.

61. Kim EY, Eisele DW, Goldberg AN, et al. Neck dissections in the United States from 2000 to 2006: volume, indications, and regionalization. Head Neck 2011; 33(6):768–73.

62. Weymuller E Jr. Matching graduate education with societal need. Laryngoscope 2005;115(2):218–22.

63. Kochhar A, Pronovost PJ, Gourin CG. Hospital-acquired conditions in head and neck cancer surgery. Laryngoscope 2013;123(7):1660–9.

64. Genther DJ, Gourin CG. The effect of hospital safety-net burden status on short-term outcomes and cost of care after head and neck cancer surgery. Arch Otolaryngol Head Neck Surg 2012;138(11):1015–22.

65. Chen AY, Fedewa S, Pavluck A, et al. Improved survival is associated with treatment at high-volume teaching facilities for patients with advanced stage laryngeal cancer. Cancer 2010;116(20):4744–52.

66. Bhattacharyya N, Abemayor E. Patterns of hospital utilization for head and neck cancer care: changing demographics. JAMA Otolaryngol Head Neck Surg 2015; 141(4):307–12.

67. Smith A, Handorf E, Arjmand E, et al. Predictors of regional Medicare expenditures for otolaryngology physician services. Laryngoscope 2017;127(6):1312–7.

68. Baker DK. Rural surgery in Canada. World J Surg 2006;30(9):1632–3.

69. Anderson RL, Anderson MA. Rural general surgery: a review of the current situation and realities from a rural community practice in Central Nebraska. Online Journal of Rural Research & Policy 2012;7(2). https://doi.org/10.4148/ojrrp.v7i2.1669.

70. Iglesias S, Kornelsen J, Woollard R, et al. Joint position paper on rural surgery and operative delivery. Can J Rural Med 2015;20(4):129–38.

71. Camilleri S. The ACA medicaid expansion, disproportionate share hospitals, and uncompensated care. Health Serv Res 2017. [Epub ahead of print].

72. Andrulis DP, Duchon LM. The changing landscape of hospital capacity in large cities and suburbs: implications for the safety net in metropolitan America. J Urban Health 2007;84(3):400–14.

Printed and bound by CPI Group (UK) Ltd, Croydon, CR0 4YY

16/10/2024

01775225-0001